Behavioral and Biochemical Issues in Substance Abuse

Behavioral and Biochemical Issues in Substance Abuse

Frank R. George, PhD
Doris Clouet, PhD
Guest Editors

Barry Stimmel, MD
Editor

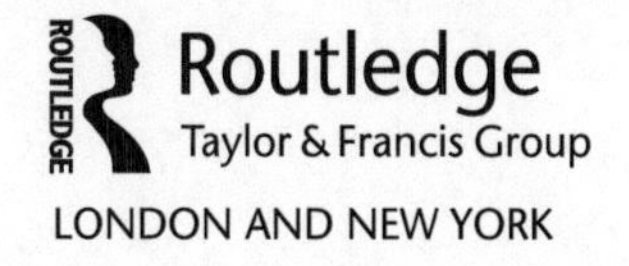

LONDON AND NEW YORK

First published 1991 by
The Haworth Press, Inc., 10 Alice Street, Binghamton, NY 13904-1580 USA

Published 2016 by Routledge
711 Third Avenue,
New York, NY 10017, USA
2 Park Square, Milton Park,
Abingdon, Oxfordshire OX14 4RN

First issued in paperback 2016

Routledge is an imprint of the Taylor & Francis Group, an informa business

Behavioral and Biochemical Issues in Substance Abuse has also been published as *Journal of Addictive Diseases*, Volume 10, Numbers 1/2 1991.

The Haworth Press, Inc., 10 Alice Street, Binghamton, NY 13904-1580 USA
EUROSPAN/Haworth, 3 Henrietta Street, London WC2E 8LU England
Haworth/ASTAM, 162-168 Parramatta Road, Stanmore, Sydney, N.S.W. 2048 Australia

Library of Congress Cataloging-in-Publication Data

Behavioral and biochemical issues in substance abuse/Frank R. George, Doris Clouet, guest editors; Barry Stimmel, editor.
p. cm.
Based on a conference held June 16-17 at Keystone, Colo. in conjunction with the 51st Annual Scientific Meeting of the Committee on Problems of Drug Dependence, Inc.
"Has also been published as Journal of addictive diseases, volume 10, numbers 1/2, 1991"—T.p.
Includes bibliographical references.
ISBN 1-56024-088-1 (alk. paper)
1. Substance abuse—Genetic aspects—Congresses. 2. Neuropsychopharmacology—Congresses. I. George, Frank Richard. II. Clouet, Doris H. III. Stimmel, Barry, 1939- . IV. Committee on Problems of Drug Dependence (U.S.). Scientific Meeting (51st : 1989 : Keystone, Colo.)
[DNLM: 1. Behavior—drug effects—congresses. 2. Substance Abuse—genetics—congresses. W1 AD432 v. 10 no. 1/2 / WM 270 B571 1989]
RC564.B4273 1990
616.86′042—dc20
DNLM/DLC
for Library of Congress

90-5325
CIP

ISBN 13: 978-1-138-98775-3 (pbk)
ISBN 13: 978-1-56024-088-4 (hbk)

Behavioral and Biochemical Issues in Substance Abuse

CONTENTS

ABOUT THE EDITORS

Frank R. George, PhD, is Senior Fellow at the National Institute on Drug Abuse Research Center, Baltimore, Maryland and Assistant Professor of Pharmacology and Toxicology in the School of Pharmacy at the University of Maryland. A behavioral geneticist and pharmacologist with fifteen years of research experience and numerous publications in the fields of alcoholism and drug abuse, Dr. George earned his doctoral degree at the University of Colorado's acclaimed institute for Behavioral Genetics and founded the intramural behavioral genetics research program of the National Institute on Drug Abuse. He is an internationally recognized leader in the area of biological risk factors in substance abuse.

Doris Clouet, PhD, has been a project officer with the National Institute on Drug Abuse, where she led the development of a strong commitment to neuroscience and genetic studies related to drug abuse. For many years she has been a widely recognized and respected neurochemist working in the biology of the brain with specialization in study of effects of drugs of abuse on the nervous system. She has authored and contributed to many papers, books, and monographs in the neurosciences, especially in the area of substance abuse.

Behavioral and Biochemical Issues in Substance Abuse

EDITORIAL

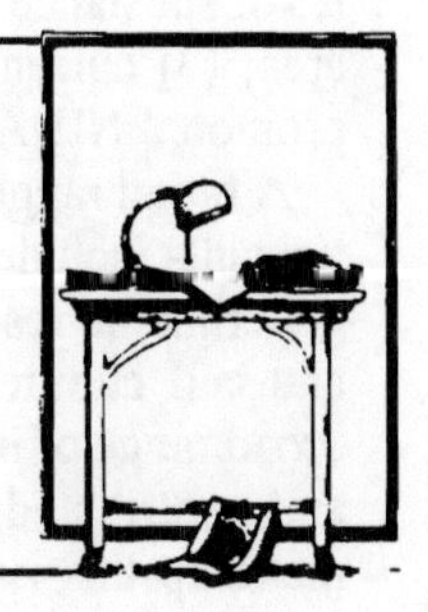

Behavioral and Biochemical Genetic Issues in Substance Abuse

For many years there has been significant interest and research within the area of biological vulnerability to alcohol abuse. However, with other abused substances, such as opiates and cocaine, historically the majority of interest and research effort has dealt with environmental and behavioral variables which contribute to substance abuse disorders. Due in part to the clear contribution of genetic factors in alcohol abuse, and data indicating genetic differences in response to many drugs in animal models of substance abuse and drug effects, the National Institute on Drug Abuse (NIDA) has increased its interest in the contribution of genetic factors and biological vulnerability to substance abuse. One result of this increased interest was the decision to organize a NIDA Technical Review conference entitled "Behavioral and Biochemical Genetic Issues in Substance Abuse." This conference was held June 16-17, 1989 at Keystone, Colorado USA, in conjunction with the annual meeting of the Committee on Problems of Drug Dependence, Inc. This meeting served several purposes: (1) it brought together investigators currently working on the genetics of substance abuse; (2) it helped to define the state of knowledge in this area; (3) current needs and future directions were discussed; and (4) it promoted NIDA's increasing interest in this area.

A broad range of interests were represented at this meeting, as the participants included NIDA administrative officers, as well as university and government researchers conducting studies involving humans, rodents and cell cultures. In addition, a number of individuals, representing a broad range of interests in substance abuse issues, attended the conference and contributed to the discussion sessions. The following papers which make up this issue of *Journal of Addictive Diseases* are based upon the presentations from this conference. Regardless of the specific methods and species used, there are some common themes and concepts which unite these papers as well as the investigators as behavioral geneticists.

Perhaps the primary concept which underlies this area is that genes can be used as independent variables. This idea forms the basis for a unique and powerful approach to biomedical research in general and to drug abuse research in particular. The understanding that genes can be used as independent variables is important for two critical reasons. The first reason is that genotype can be systematically manipulated or varied, which allows for the estimation of genetic contributions to various dependent measures, such as behavioral responses to drugs. The second reason is that genotype can be controlled or held constant. When genotype is held constant, then any variation found in a dependent measure is presumably due to environmental effects. Therefore, the ideal way to study genetic factors is to thoroughly control for environmental variation, and the ideal way to study environmental factors is to completely control for genetic variation.

One overall consensus reached at this conference was that, in terms of non-alcohol related substance abuse studies, environmental effects have been explored and controlled for in an excellent manner, but genetic factors are very poorly understood and controlled, and that this is an area where further progress is important to our understanding of both genetic as well as environmental factors involved in substance abuse.

Genetic variation in response to drugs can be used as a powerful research tool. In terms of animal models, genetic selection for divergent phenotypes related to drug effects is an important method which is being effectively used in studying alcohol, and is now being adopted into a growing number of projects related to mechanisms of non-alcohol drugs, such as opiates, nicotine, cocaine and benzodiazepines. The paper by Andrew Smolen and Michael Marks[1] describes the use of selective breeding paradigms to produce novel lines of mice which differ maximally in Y-maze activating response to nicotine, and additional independent lines of mice which differ in activating response to cocaine. Initial findings show clear evidence of heritability for these responses, and early progress is encouraging. John Belknap[2] presented elegant autoradiographic data related to his selective breeding project for high vs. low antinociceptive response to levorphanol. His mice currently differ by seven-fold in this measure of analgesia, and he showed that these mice show significant differences in density of dorsal raphe nucleus mu receptor sites. Edward Gallaher and coworkers[3] have developed selectively bred lines of mice which differ substantially in response to diazepam when using rotorod stability as the phenotype. Interestingly, these mice do not differ in diazepam-induced seizure protection, suggesting that the anticonvulsant and muscle relaxant effects of diazepam are associated with different biological pathways. The paper by Janice Froehlich and Ting-Kai Li[4] reviews the status of the widely recognized alcohol-preferring and alcohol non-preferring rat lines. Studying the procedures used in their successful alcohol studies can aid in the development of appropriate selective breeding studies for divergent intake of non-alcohol drugs of abuse.

Another method which holds great potential in the study of substance abuse involves the use of Recombinant Inbred (RI) strains of rodents. The report by Tamara Phillips and coworkers[5] provides an excellent introduction to the use of RI strains in identifying major gene effects, mapping traits to particular chromosomes, and in studying genetic relationships among different traits. The authors then describe the status of their own work using these methods in studying possible major gene effects moderating alcohol or morphine intake. Jeanne Wehner and coworkers[6] discuss the use of RI strains as it relates to the development of the LSXSS RI strains, which have recently been derived from the well known LS and SS selectively bred lines. These authors show how these LSXSS RI mice have already been used to estimate the number of genes involved in mediating neurosensitivity to ethanol, and how they are being used to study biological mechanisms associated with responses to ethanol.

A third pharmacogenetic method used by several of the participating investigators involves comparing responses on various behavioral and/or biochemical phenotypes across multiple inbred strains to obtain an estimate of the relationship, or correlation, among the traits under study. For example, the report by Allan Collins and Michael Marks[7] describes their studies examining the relationships among several behavioral and physiological responses to nicotine with numbers of brain nicotinic receptors in various brain regions. These authors also present preliminary findings suggesting the presence of genetic differences in nicotine intake in mice.

This idea of genetic differences in drug-taking behaviors is being studied in a growing number of laboratories. The report by Frank George[8] summarizes the work by him and his associates on genetic contributions to alcohol, opiate and cocaine self-administration and home cage drinking. The findings are intriguing in that they suggest possible common determinants of reinforcement from these different abused substances. These studies are complemented by the work presented in the two papers by John Carney, Thomas Seale and their colleagues.[9,10] These investigators present pharmacogenetic data on a number of animal models of response to cocaine as well as possible reinforcement from cocaine, using nonself-administration models such as conditioned place preference. Taken together, these three reports[8-10] present an important direction in the field as they will hopefully result in a better defined and greater consensus on what is meant by "drug reinforced behavior".

Across all of the behavioral studies it is important to keep in mind the specific phenotypes being measured, and their specific advantages and disadvantages. The paper by Richard Meisch[11] addresses methodological issues in two behavioral areas critical to our understanding of substance abuse behavior, namely drug-reinforced behavior and drug discrimination. For example, it is important to distinguish between the study of initiation of self-administration or discrimination and the maintenance of these behaviors, as different methods will be involved, and the behaviors may likely be mediated by dissimilar mechanisms.

Much of the work in the reports at this meeting has as one ultimate goal defining those underlying biochemical traits associated with behavioral responses to drugs, especially drug self-administration. Mary Ritz[12] presents findings as well as important methodological and conceptual concerns relevant to the conduct of biochemical genetic studies. One important question raised is how much effect does one gene have on a receptor. We know that there are a number of significant single gene effects on behavior, but how do single genetic variants affect receptor structure or regulation? For example, as much as the dopamine transporter site appears to be highly associated with the reinforcing effects of cocaine, she shows that there are no significant differences in ligand affinity or number for either the dopamine transporter site or D1 or D2 receptor sites across rat strains that differ in self-administration of cocaine.

At this meeting the status and future of human genetic studies on substance abuse were also discussed. Roy Pickens and Dace Svikis present reviews of findings from human adoption and twin studies of substance abuse.[13,14] Dr. Pickens stresses the complementary nature of human and animal model studies arguing effectively for the importance of both levels of investigation.[13] Dr. Svikis examines several methodological assumptions and procedures important in the appropriate conduct of human genetic studies in substance abuse.[14]

A specific issue in human studies discussed at the meeting is specific population prevalence, an issue raised by both Drs. Pickens and Svikis in their presentations. For example, when studying twins reared apart, one twin may be reared in a region with high prevalence of cocaine use while the other twin is reared in a region with low cocaine use. Under these conditions, it may be difficult to assess whether non-concordance for cocaine abuse is the result of a lack of genetic influence on this trait, or due to confounding environmental factors such as drug access.

An exciting possibility in substance abuse research which is just beginning to emerge is the use of cell culture studies as presented in the work by John Madden and Arthur Falek.[15] These authors show that nonneuronal cells can react directly with opiates *in vitro*, which has significant impact on metabolic processes within these cells. This work may lead to studies with twins or families which would involve not just psychosocial or behavioral measures, but also the attainment of peripheral cell populations that can be cultured and studied in terms of specific receptor populations. This would provide a method for determining markers and risk for substance abuse disorders.

Together, the findings from this meeting, whether based upon human, rodent or cellular studies, indicate that there are large genetic differences in response to abused substances. Animal models are being effectively utilized to examine drug mechanisms and correlated traits, while at the human level emerging findings indicate a need for further studies to identify specific biological factors which contribute to individual variation in responses to drugs and in the development of substance abuse disorders.

We sincerely thank all of the participants for contributing to an exciting, interesting and informative meeting. It is hoped that this meeting and these papers will contribute significantly towards a greater understanding of the mechanisms of action of abused substances, and will aid in determining the extent of biological vulnerability and risk for the development of substance abuse disorders in humans.

Frank R. George, PhD
Doris Clouet, PhD

REFERENCES

1. Smolen A, Marks MJ. Genetic selections for nicotine and cocaine sensitivity in mice. Adv Alcohol Subst Abuse. 1991; 10(1-2).

2. Belknap JK. Where are the mu receptors that mediate opioid analgesia?: An autoradiographic study in the HAR and LAR selection lines. Adv Alcohol Subst Abuse. 1991; 10(1-2).

3. Gallaher EJ, Gionet SE, Feller DJ. Behavioral and neurochemical studies in diazepam-sensitive and -resistant mice. Adv Alcohol Subst Abuse. 1991; 10(1-2).

4. Froehlich JC, Li T-K. Animal models for the study of alcoholism: Utility of selected lines. Adv Alcohol Subst Abuse. 1991; 10(1-2).

5. Phillips TJ, Belknap JK, Crabbe JC. Use of recombinant inbred strains to access vulnerability to drug abuse at the genetic level. Adv Alcohol Subst Abuse. 1991; 10(1-2).

6. Wehner JM, Pounder JI, Bowers BJ. The use of recombinant inbred strains to study mechanisms of drug action. Adv Alcohol Subst Abuse. 1991; 10(1-2).

7. Collins AC, Marks MJ. Progress towards the development of animal models of smoking-related behaviors. Adv Alcohol Subst Abuse. 1991; 10(1-2).

8. George FR. Is there a common biological basis for reinforcement from alcohol and other drugs? Adv Alcohol Subst Abuse. 1991; 10(1-2).

9. Seale TW, Carney JM. Genetics determinants of susceptibility to the rewarding and other behavioral actions of psychomotor stimulants. Adv Alcohol Subst Abuse. 1991; 10(1-2).

10. Carney JM, Cheng M-S, Wu C, Seale TW. Issues surrounding the assessment of the genetic determinants of drugs as reinforcing stimuli. Adv Alcohol Subst Abuse. 1991; 19(1-2).

11. Meisch RA. Establishment of drug discrimination and drug reinforcement in different animal strains: Some methodological issues. Adv Alcohol Subst Abuse. 1991; 10(1-2).

12. Ritz MC. Biochemical genetic differences in vulnerability to drug effects: Is statistically significant always physiologically important and vice versa. Adv Alcohol Subst Abuse. 1991; 10(1-2).

13. Pickens RW, Svikis DS. Genetic influences in human substance abuse. Adv Alcohol Subst Abuse. 1991; 10(1-2).

14. Svikis DS, Pickens, RW. Methodological issues in genetic studies of human substance abuse. Adv Alcohol Subst Abuse. 1991; 10(1-2).

15. Madden JJ, Falek A. The use of nonneuronal cells as *in vitro* model systems for studying the genetics of opiate abuse. Adv Alcohol Subst Abuse. 1991; 10(1-2).

Genetic Selections for Nicotine and Cocaine Sensitivity in Mice

Andrew Smolen, PhD
Michael J. Marks, PhD

SUMMARY. We are using selective breeding to develop lines of mice which differ maximally in their responses to nicotine, and independent lines of mice which differ maximally in their responses to cocaine. The foundation population was the genetically heterogeneous HS mice. On day 1, baseline (saline injected) activity of each mouse was measured in an automated Y-maze over 3 minutes. On day 2, animals were tested for sensitivity to nicotine (0.75 mg/kg) in the same apparatus. A residual score, calculated from the regression of nicotine scores on saline scores for the whole population, was calculated for each animal. The most severely affected mice (lowest residual scores) were mated to form duplicate Nicotine-Depressed lines; the most stimulated mice (highest residual scores) were mated to form duplicate Nicotine-Activated lines. A random sampling of individuals was chosen without regard to residual scores for production of duplicate Control lines. Duplicate lines of mice activated and depressed by cocaine are being produced in an analogous fashion using 50 mg/kg cocaine as the test dose. Successful selective breeding for a drug-related trait provides clear evidence of a heritable component for that trait. These selected lines of mice will ultimately be used to study hypotheses involving genetic control of response to these drugs.

Andrew Smolen and Michael J. Marks are affiliated with the Institute for Behavioral Genetics and Drug Abuse Research Center, Campus Box 447, University of Colorado, Boulder, CO 80309-0447. Correspondence may be addressed to Dr. Smolen at the above address.

The authors wish to thank Ms. Robin Richeson for her excellent technical assistance, Ms. Rebecca G. Miles for editorial assistance and Drs. Norman D. Henderson and John C. DeFries for many useful discussions.

This project is supported by a grant from the National Institute on Drug Abuse, DA05131.

The role of genetic factors in influencing drug responses in animals can be studied using inbred strains, recombinant inbred strains, heterogeneous populations or lines of animals genetically selected to differ maximally for a trait of interest.[1] Each of these approaches has been used to some extent, but the overwhelming majority of genetic investigations has concentrated on inbred strain comparisons. We are in the process of developing lines of mice which are differentially sensitive to nicotine, and independent lines which are differentially sensitive to cocaine. In this paper we will discuss some of the advantages of using selective breeding for differential drug sensitivity, outline some of the considerations which should be addressed in designing and implementing such a study, and provide a brief description of the results obtained from testing of the foundation population.

Inbred strains, which have been most widely used in genetic studies, are produced by mating close relatives, generally brother-sister, over numerous (20 minimum) generations to obtain fixation and homozygosity of virtually all genetic loci. One member of an inbred strain can be considered to be a genetic replicate of all other members of that strain. The major advantage of inbred strains is their relative constancy over time. Members of an inbred strain tested today for a particular biochemical or behavioral trait are very nearly the same as members of that strain tested several years ago on the same measurement. If several inbred strains reared in the same laboratory are found to differ in response to a drug, this is taken as *prima facie* evidence for a genetic basis for the difference. A second advantage of using inbred strains for genetic studies is the availability of literally hundreds of strains. A screen of a modest number of these strains can often reveal two which differ markedly in a trait of interest. These strains can then be used to investigate potential genetic regulation of the trait of interest using methods such as classical cross (comparison of 2 inbred strains, their F_1 hybrids, and F_2 and backcross generations) and diallel (comparison of several inbred strains and all possible F_1 crosses) analyses. Thirdly, inbred strains are often well characterized for a number of biochemical and behavioral traits. This can be of advantage in the initial choice of strains to screen or to assess potential confounding characteristics of a strain.

The genetic homogeneity of inbred strains, which may be advantageous when comparing animals across time and laboratories, is a marked disadvantage when one is interested in differences between individuals or correlations between two or more responses. The total phenotypic variance of a population, V_P, can be described as the sum of its genotypic variance, V_G, its environmental variance, V_E, and variance due to possible interactions between genotype and environment, $V_{(G \times E)}$: $V_P = V_G + V_E + V_{(G \times E)}$.[2,3] Since fixation of alleles reduces genetic variance within strains to nearly zero, inbred strains are of limited value in studies where correlational analysis is to be employed. Two traits may correlate highly among inbred strains because of chance fixation of alleles during inbreeding, and may not imply a cause-effect relationship.

Recombinant Inbred (RI) strains offer a more sophisticated approach to studying genetic mechanisms underlying differences between the two inbreds. RI strains are produced by mating 2 inbred strains to produce the F_1 generation. The F_1 animals are then mated to produce the F_2 generation. This is a segregating population in which individuals may have different alleles at any locus where the original inbred strains differed. The purpose of the F_2 generation in producing RI strains is to shuffle the alleles of the parental strains randomly among individuals and to break up linkages between loci. Pairs of male and female F_2 siblings are then chosen to produce multiple (40 or more) RI strains, which are considered inbred after 20 generations of full-sib matings. The resulting RI lines contain random pairings of the genetic information at each locus from the parental lines. The major use of RI strains is to test for single gene effects using strain distribution patterns as described in another paper in this volume. The major disadvantage to RI strains is that the genetic information they provide is limited by the degree to which the parental strains differed. They are, however, powerful genetic tools which have been underused for studies of drug effects.

Heterogeneous populations offer another method for studying genetic effects on drug responses. In this case the genotypic variance of the population is non-zero, and differences among individuals is due to genetic as well as environmental factors. A genetically heterogeneous population is of much more utility in correlational studies than are inbred strains. In this case the contribution of the genotypic co-variance to the correlation is much less likely to be fortuitous; thus, one may undertake to investigate genetic mechanisms underlying correlations between two measurements.

There are comparatively few heterogeneous stocks of laboratory animals for use in pharmacogenetic research. One is often limited to lines such as Swiss-Webster mice or Wistar or Sprague-Dawley rats. These animals are generally regarded as being "outbred" and therefore heterogeneous to some extent, but in most cases their history is simply not known. Depending on the source, these lines may be considerably inbred, which is also indicated by the fact that all of these lines are albino (a recessive allele). In contrast, McClearn and coworkers[4] constructed a heterogeneous stock of mice (HS) by intercrossing eight inbred strains. The HS stock is maintained by randomly mating 40 pairs of animals with no common grandparental ancestry each generation. These animals represent a truly heterogeneous population and have been used for a wide range of studies; however, their main utility has been as the foundation population for a number of genetic selection studies.

The use of a heterogeneous foundation population for selecting lines of animals with large behavioral differences was first demonstrated by Tolman[5] in his studies of maze learning in rats. Tolman's two-generation selection study formed the foundation for the classical work of Tryon[6] who succeeded in establishing maze-bright and maze-dull lines of rats with non-overlapping distributions after only seven generations of selection. This well-known selection experiment was in turn a prototype for a number of other selection experiments for such diverse characteristics as motor activity[7] and emotionality in rats,[8] and body weight,[9] susceptibility to audiogenic seizures,[10] litter size and lactation,[11] open-field activity,[12] acoustic priming-induced seizures[13] and nest building[14] in mice. The utility of selective breeding in establishing phenotypes for the pharmacological investigations of drug responses is exemplified by selection studies for ethanol preference in rats,[15,16] acute response to ethanol,[17] severity of the ethanol withdrawal syndrome,[18,19] hypothermic effects of ethanol,[20] differential ethanol-induced locomotor activity,[21] sensitivity to diazepam[22] and sensitivity to opiate antinociception[23] in mice.

A successful selective breeding program for a drug-related phenotype provides clear evidence of a heritable component for that phenotype, and the resulting animals may be very useful for the study of the mechanisms through which the genes exert their influence upon the phenotype. In order for a selection experiment to be successful, there must be recognizable individual differences within the population. Some of this variation is due to environmental factors, but this source of variation is not heritable and does not influence response to selection pressure. In a properly designed selection experiment, differences among lines will be due at least in part to changes in frequencies of alleles which determine, directly or indirectly, that phenotype. Thus, a correlated response to selection implies a genetic correlation with the selected character. Selected lines are, therefore, effective for testing hypotheses concerning drug actions, since differences between the lines, be they behavioral (e.g., drug self administrarion), physiological (e.g., effects on heart rate) or biochemical (e.g., regulation of neurotransmitter receptors), are likely to be related to the mechanism of action of the drug. For example, if the activity of a neurotransmitter system thought to be involved in drug sensitivity is found to be the same in both lines, that system probably does not mediate that response.

Another advantage of a selection study is that the response of the selected lines to the selection criterion often exceeds the maximum differences in the foundation population. This has been well demonstrated by the long-sleep (LS)/short-sleep (SS) mouse selection by McClearn and Kakihana,[17] and the selection for open-field activity in mice by DeFries and coworkers.[12,24,25] Both studies resulted in selected lines with means which far exceeded the range of responses in foundation population. Thus, by changing allelic frequencies by selective breeding, it is possible to produce animals with responses exceeding those of natural populations. This can be utilized to great advantage when testing hypotheses concerning drug action.

In this paper we will outline our approach to using selective breeding to develop lines of mice which differ maximally in their responses to nicotine, and independent lines of mice which differ maximally in their responses to cocaine. The availability of these selectively bred lines will enable us to examine hypotheses involving genetic control of responses to these drugs.

METHODS

The goal of a bi-directional selection study is to accumulate alleles involved in sensitivity to a drug in the sensitive lines and alleles involved in drug resistance in the resistant lines while leaving all other alleles randomly distributed. A properly designed genetic selection experiment must include certain features at its inception to insure that possible chance associations between spurious parameters and the selected phenotype are kept to a minimum.[24-28] Since response to selection is a function of the amount of additive genetic variance present in a population, it is important to maintain genetic variance within the selected lines. This may be readily accomplished by starting with a population as heterogeneous as possible, and by using as large a number of mating pairs per line as feasible to insure that inbreeding within the selected line is kept to a minimum. In a randomly mated population of mice, a closed line consisting of 10 mating pairs will have a coefficient of inbreeding of less than 1.5% per generation,[2] which is generally considered to be acceptable.

A second important consideration in a selection experiment is the inclusion of a contemporaneous, unselected control line containing a number of mating pairs equal to the selected lines. A control line is useful to evaluate effects of possible intergeneration environmental fluctuations and effects of possible inbreeding in the selected lines. The high and low lines may each be measured by their deviation from the control mean; thus, any asymmetry of response to selection (either direct or correlated) may be ascertained.

A third critical feature which must be included in a selection study is replication. Since large intergeneration variability is often found in a selection study, especially early on, replicated lines allow for the assessment of the generality of response to selection. Replication is especially important to test hypotheses concerning mechanisms. Chance changes in frequencies of alleles unrelated to the character under selection will often occur. If replicates of the lines are available, any hypothesis of genetic association may be tested immediately. Since chance associations between characters unrelated to the phenotype under selection would not be expected to occur in both replicates, a correlated response found in both replicates is likely to be due to causal factors.

A fourth feature which should be included in the design of a selection experiment is bi-directional selection: the contemporaneous selection of lines more and less sensitive than the foundation population. Selecting high and low lines simultaneously maximizes the potential to produce large differences between the lines. This also requires that the test used allows for scores which can go higher or lower than those in the foundation population.

Our selection studies contain each of the features listed above. The foundation population was the genetically heterogeneous HS mice. Genetic heterogeneity is being retained by maintaining 10 mating pairs for each selected line. We are producing replicated lines of mice which show (1) reduced (depressed) locomotor activity (compared to saline baseline) following nicotine administration (Nicotine Depressed "ND1," "ND2"); (2) increased (activated) locomotor activity following nicotine administration (Nicotine Activated, "NA1," "NA2"); (3) reduced locomotor activity following cocaine administration (Cocaine Depressed "CD1," "CD2"); and (4) increased locomotor activity following cocaine administration (Cocaine Activated, "CA1," "CA2"). Moreover, replicated unselected control lines ("C1," "C2") are being produced. One advantage of performing the selection studies for nicotine and cocaine simultaneously is that the same replicate control lines can be used for both selection studies, thus saving animals and space. We are performing bidirectional selection for each drug using a locomotor test that allows for both increased and decreased activity. Finally, we are employing within-family selection which minimizes inbreeding. For example, in the resistant lines, the most resistant male and female from each of 10 litters are selected for mating. These animals will be mated randomly to produce the next generation.

Experimental Animals

The foundation population for the selection studies was the Heterogeneous Stock mice developed by McClearn and coworkers.[4] The selected lines were derived from 40 families of HS mice currently on hand. All mice are housed in the Specific Pathogen Free (SPF) facility of the Institute for Behavioral Genetics (IBG). Mice are kept in a constant temperature, constant humidity environment with a 12-hr light cycle (lights on 0700-1900). and are allowed free access to food (Wayne Sterilizable Lab Blox) and water.

Drugs

The drugs we are studying are nicotine and cocaine. Concurrent selection studies on these drugs will allow us to study potential commonalties between nicotine and cocaine directly. It has been suggested that both drugs (and amphetamine, as well) exert at least some of their effects by causing the release of, or inhibition of, reuptake of catechol- and indoleamines, either of which would result in increased synaptic concentrations of biogenic amines. The possibility that cross-tolerance (or sensitivity) might occur between them is suggested by studies which have shown that smokers are often unable to distinguish between intravenously administered cocaine or nicotine.[29]

Y-Maze Activity

The Y-maze measures voluntary locomotor activity. The apparatus is an enclosed red Plexiglas Y-maze 25 cm × 25 cm × 10 cm, divided into six areas (two per arm) by photoelectric beams. Crossing of a beam activates a counter which accumulates the number of beams crossed during the 3-min. test. The number of beams crossed is recorded as the total activity score. An additional set of photoelectric beams mounted 5 cm above the floor of the apparatus is used to count the number of rearings. Number of rearings is measured as a correlated response to selection. Testing is conducted between 1000 and 1500 hours.

Body Temperature

The assessment of the effects of drugs on body temperature is a relatively easy and reliable test in a constant temperature environment such as the SPF laboratory at IBG. Rectal temperature is measured using a Thermalert THS probe (Bailey Instruments). This probe equilibrates within 5 sec. and measures temperature to the nearest 0.1°. Body temperature is being measured as a correlated response to selection.

Regression Residuals as the Selection Criterion

Since we are interested in drug-induced activity, the simplest method would be to administer the drug to the mouse, measure its activity level, and then choose the most active for the high lines and the least active for the low lines. That system, however, does not take into account the animal's baseline (saline-injected) activity level, and it is possible that we would be selecting on the basis of overall, not specifically drug-induced, activity. In order to select for drug induced response, some method of controlling for basal activity should be used. Difference scores (drug minus saline) have commonly been used for this purpose. There are, however, a number of problems with difference scores, the most serious being that they are often found to be negatively correlated with baseline measurements.[30] In contrast, deviations from regression, more commonly called regression residuals, correct for any correlation between pretreatment and posttreatment measurements.[30,31] Regression residuals represent the difference between drug response predicted from the saline vs. drug regression line and the actual response measured.

Comparisons between difference scores and regression residual scores can best be seen with a simple, model data set as shown in Table 1. The regression equation is calculated for the whole population with observed (measured) saline score (S_i, column 1) on the x-axis and observed (measured) drug score (D_i, column 2) on the y-axis. For this example, expected drug score = 2 + [0.2 * (saline score)]. Each animal's saline score is substituted into the equation, and an expected drug score ($\hat{D}_i$) is calculated for each individual (column 3). The regression residual for that individual (denoted D_i - $\hat{D}_i$) is simply the difference between the observed drug score and the expected drug score (column 4). These data are graphically represented in Figure 1. The difference score (D_i - S_i) for each individual is tabulated in column 5. Some properties of difference scores and regression residuals are shown by the correlations listed at the bottom of Table 1.

The correlation coefficient, *r*, and the regression coefficient, b (the slope of the regression line), are both 0.2 for this example (equation 1).

TABLE 1. Comparison of Deviations from Regression with Difference Scores

Saline Score (observed)	Drug Score (observed)	Drug Score (expected)	Regession Deviation Score	Difference Score
S_i	D_i	$\hat{D}_i$	$D_i - \hat{D}_i$	$D_i - S_i$
3	1	2.6	-1.6	-2
4	4	2.8	+1.2	0
5	5	3.0	+2.0	0
6	2	3.2	-1.2	-4
7	3	3.4	-0.4	-4

(1) Correlation and regression coefficients obtained from the plot of saline scores vs. drug scores:

$$b_{DS} = 0.2, \qquad r_{DS} = 0.2$$

(2) Regression equation obtained from the plot of saline scores vs. drug scores:

$$\hat{D}_i = \bar{D} + b_{DS}\,(S_i - \bar{S}) = 2 + 0.2\,S_i$$

(3) Correlation between difference scores and saline scores:

$$r_{(D_i - S_i)(S_i)} = -0.63$$

(4) Correlation between residual scores and saline scores:

$$r_{(D_i - \hat{D}_i)(S_i)} = 0$$

(5) Correlation between difference scores and drug scores:

$$r_{(D_i - S_i)(D_i)} = 0.63$$

(6) Correlation between residual scores and drug scores:

$$r_{(D_i - \hat{D}_i)(D_i)} = 0.98$$

FIGURE 1. Correlation between saline scores and drug scores for the sample data shown in Table 1. Observed scores are indicated by the open circles, expected scores calculated from the regression equation are indicated by the closed circles. The regression residuals (difference between observed and expected scores) are indicated by the vertical bars.

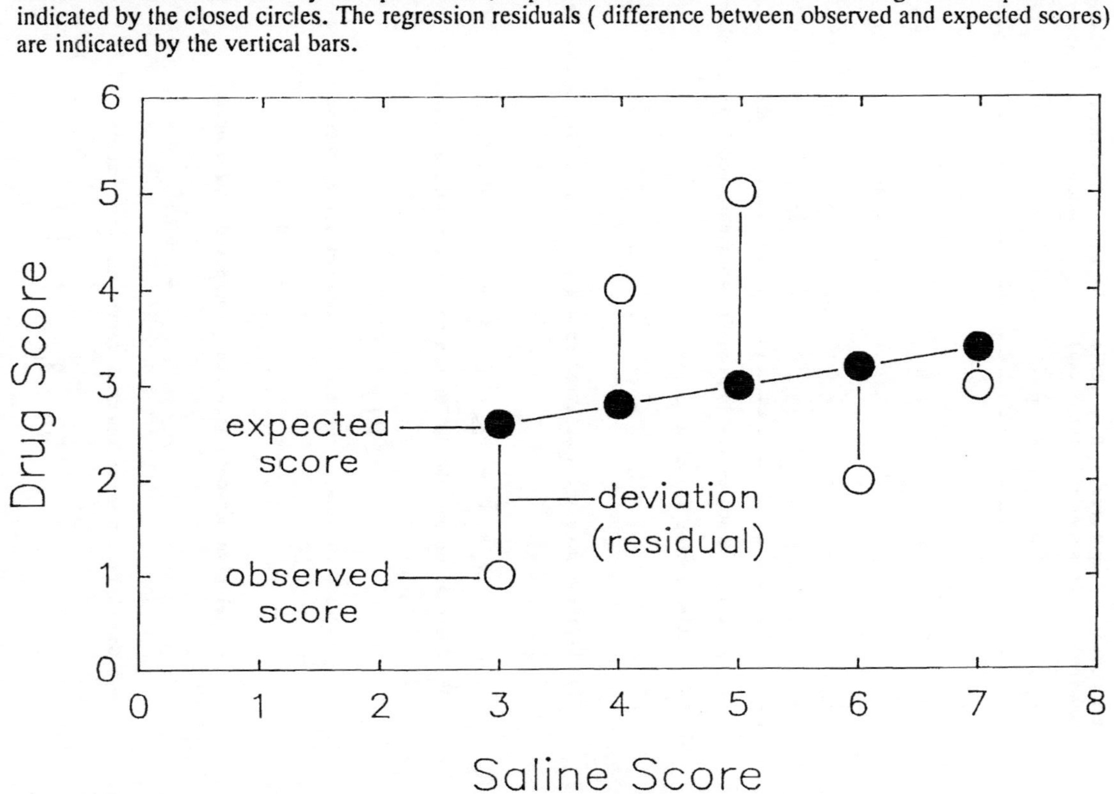

Equality of these two parameter estimates was chosen for convenience; it is not necessary in the general case. Equation (3) is the correlation between the difference scores and the baseline saline scores. It is negative and greater (−0.63) than the correlation between the original drug and saline scores (0.20). This illustrates one of the most serious drawbacks to difference scores: they are still correlated with baseline scores, but the sign is now reversed. Equation (4) is the correlation between residual scores and saline scores. This correlation is zero, indicating that residual scores are independent of baseline scores—clearly an advantage. Equation (5) is the correlation between difference scores and drug scores. It is large and positive (0.63), showing that difference scores can be very good measures of drug-induced activity. However, equation (6), the correlation between regression residuals and drug scores, is nearly unity, indicating even better agreement between residuals and drug scores than was found for difference scores—again, an advantage.

These relationships allow us to draw several conclusions about the utility of difference scores and regression residuals as measures of drug effects: (1) Difference scores can be strongly influenced by baseline scores, often in the direction opposite to that found in the original data, whereas residual scores are not. Regression residuals compensate well for pretreatment effects, whereas difference scores may not. (2) Both difference scores and regression residuals are more highly correlated with drug scores than are baseline scores, however, residuals are more highly correlated with drug scores than are difference scores. (3) Residuals are generally more reliable than difference scores (we will comment more on this result in another communication). (4) The relative advantage of residuals over difference scores becomes less as the correlation between saline and drug scores increases. For highly correlated traits they may be nearly equal, but at no point are difference scores superior to residuals. For moderately correlated traits ($r < 0.5$), residual scores appear to be superior to difference scores.

We do not wish to suggest, however, that the use of difference scores in selection experiments is in any way erroneous, only that residuals may often be superior. Crabbe[32] reviewed his selection criteria using both change scores and regression residuals and found that the same animals would have been chosen over 75% of the time using either method. Clearly, both methods have validity in assessing drug responses, but since regression residuals are uncorrelated with saline baseline, and highly correlated with drug scores, each animal's baseline activity is accounted for, and drug-induced activity is emphasized to the maximum extent. The net result of using regression residuals is that one is likely to make progress in selection more rapidly. Since the use of regression residuals has theoretical, as well as practical, advantages over change scores, it was the method we decided to use.

For a selection study, choosing animals on the basis of difference scores is easy to understand since one simply subtracts the saline score from the drug score to obtain the difference score. Animals with greatest difference are most sensitive to the drug, and are chosen for the sensitive lines; those with the least difference are resistant to the drug, and are chosen for the resistant lines. Residuals operate the same way, except that the animals are chosen on the basis of the distance of their drug scores from the regression line (expected drug score) as indicated in Figure 1. In this case the most sensitive animals are either very close to or below the line (depending on the scale), and the least sensitive are above the regression line. For our selection studies the residual scores are of approximately the same magnitude and of the same sign as the difference scores (negative for the animals with depressed drug-induced activities, and positive for the animals with stimulated drug-induced activities). The major difference between the use of difference scores or residual scores, then, is what is subtracted from the drug score: saline score for the difference, expected drug score for the residual.

Selective Breeding for Sensitivity to Nicotine

The foundation population for the nicotine selection study was 417 male and female mice from the first litter of generation 43 obtained from 40 families of HS mice. Mice were tested for sensitivity to nicotine at 85 ± 15 days of age. On day one mice were injected intraperitoneally (i.p.) with saline (0.01 ml/g body weight). Five minutes after injection the mice were placed in a Y-maze and their total activity and number of rears were measured over the next 3 min. Fifteen minutes after injection (7 min after completion of the Y-maze test). rectal temperature was measured. Mice were then returned to their home cage. On day two each mouse was injected with nicotine, 0.75 mg/kg i.p. in saline (0.01 ml/g body weight), and their activity in the Y-maze and body temperature measured as on day one. The timing of the test and selection of nicotine dose were based on a number of preliminary experiments which we will briefly summarize. Maximum effect of nicotine on Y-maze activity occurs 5 min after intraperitoneal injection, and maximum effect on body temperature occurs at 15 min, which are the times we are using for this selection study. We chose a dose of nicotine, 0.75 mg/kg, high enough to observe decrements in activity in mice, but also low enough to be able to pick out those individuals which would be stimulated by nicotine.

Ten males and ten females were chosen at random (without regard to residual scores) from the entire population before the most nicotine-activated and most nicotine-depressed mice were selected, and these animals were mated at random to form one of the Control Lines, C1. This ensures that the control lines have a chance of containing very activated and very depressed animals, which is important in producing a truly random population for the phenotype undergoing selection. The replicate Control Line, C2, was produced during derivation of the cocaine selected lines (below). The Nicotine-Activated and Nicotine-Depressed lines were formed from the mice remaining after the Control Line mice were removed. The 20 males and 20 females with activities most depressed by nicotine (animals whose residuals were numerically most negative) were mated at random to form Selected Generation 1 (S_1) of the two Nicotine-Depressed Lines (ND1 and ND2). The two Nicotine Activated Lines, NA1 and NA2, were constructed in an analogous fashion from the 20 males and 20 females with activities most stimulated by nicotine (animals whose residuals were numerically most positive). No more than two individuals from each of the 40 HS families were included in a single line. From this point on the lines are closed. That is, all matings for ND1, for example, will come only from families within ND1.

Each line is maintained by within-family selection, which means that each family will be represented in each generation. Litters are weaned at 23 ± 2 days of age. Weanlings are housed with like-sex litrermates (2-5 per cage) until tested at 60 ± 5 days of age. The S_1 litters will be tested for nicotine sensitivity as described above on two consecutive days. S_1 animals will be selected for mating to produce Selected Generation 2 (S_2) on the basis of their regression residuals. For the low activity lines (ND1 and ND2), for example, the male and female in each S_1 litter with the greatest nicotine-induced depression of Y-maze activity will be chosen for mating to produce the next generation. These animals will be mated at random to form the 10 mating pairs for S_2. The most activated male and female from each litter will be chosen as breeders for S_2 of NA1 and NA2. The control lines are tested in the same manner as the selected lines. One male and one female is chosen at random from each litter without regard to their residual score, and mated randomly to form the second generation of control animals.

Selective Breeding for Sensitivity to Cocaine

The cocaine selection study is being performed in a manner analogous to the nicotine selection study outlined above. The foundation population for the cocaine selection study was 392 male and female mice from third litters of generation 43 obtained from 40 families of HS mice. Mice were tested for sensitivity to cocaine using the Y-maze test. They were given saline on day one and cocaine (50 mg/kg) on day two. Time between injection and activity testing was 30 min. Rectal temperature was measured 15 min after injection. From preliminary experiments we found that the maximum effect of cocaine on Y-maze activity and body temperature occurred at these times. The fact that both drugs had maximum effect on temperature at 15 min was coincidental. The dose of cocaine, 50 mg/kg, was chosen so that we would be able to detect both stimulation and depression of activity, and was arrived at following dose-response studies in a variety of inbred strains and selected lines of mice.

Derivation of the Cocaine-Depressed and Cocaine-Activated lines was accomplished as described for the nicotine selection study above. A random sampling of individuals was mated to form the second Control Line, C2. Thus, one control line was started along with the nicotine selected lines, and one along with the cocaine selected lines two months later, so that any potential time and litter effects between the nicotine and cocaine studies will be accommodated.

All procedures used in this project received prior review and approval by the University of Colorado Animal Care and Use Committee as being consistent with USPHS standards of humane care and treatment of laboratory animals.

RESULTS AND DISCUSSION

In order for a selection study to be successful, a wide range of individual differences must be evident in the foundation population. Figure 2 shows the correlation between saline activity scores and nicotine activity scores for all 417 mice tested for nicotine sensitivity. Data were combined across sex because no significant difference between the sexes was found. There was a large range in both saline baseline and nicotine-induced activity scores. We observed nicotine-induced stimulation as well as depression, indicating that the dosage was well suited to screen the HS mice for differential sensitivity to nicotine. The wide range of activity shows that the HS population is a suitable one from which to select for differential

FIGURE 2. Correlation between control Y-maze activity and activity following administration of 0.75 mg/kg nicotine in 417 male and female HS mice.

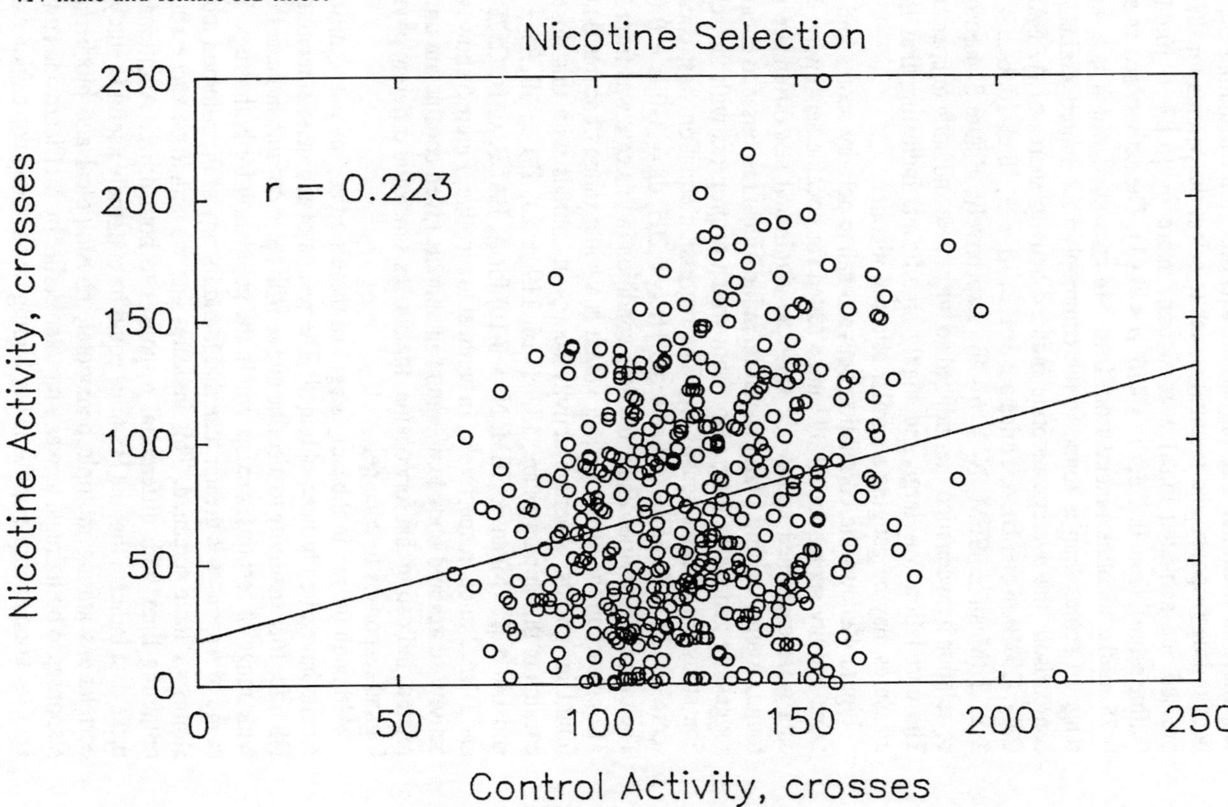

responses to nicotine. The regression equation (for calculating the expected drug response and residual scores to select the parents for the depressed and activated lines) was: nicotine score = 18.87 + [0.447 * (saline score)] (r = 0.223, df = 415, $p < 0.01$). The activity scores after 0.75 mg/kg nicotine ranged from 0 to 248 crossings, which is a wider range of scores than is found in the commonly used inbred strains. For comparison, the average nicotine induced activity scores of A, BALB, C3H, C57BL/6 and DBA/2 mice are 3 ± 2, 10 ± 5, 28 ± 10, 6 ± 4 and 2 ± 2 (Mean ± SEM, N = 6 - 9), respectively. Figure 3 shows the correlation between nicotine-induced activity score and body temperature. The correlation was large and highly significant, indicating that these measures may be gauging a similar effect of nicotine.

Figure 4 shows the correlation between saline activity scores and cocaine activity scores for all 392 mice tested for cocaine sensitivity. The data were combined across sex since no significant sex difference was found. Again, we find a large variation in individual responses to cocaine, suggesting genetic heterogeneity from which to progress with the selection study for cocaine sensitivity. The regression equation was: cocaine score = 122 + [0.358 * (saline score)] (r = 0.205, df = 390, $p < 0.01$). The range of activities under the drug condition in this case was from 1 to 312 crosses in the 3-min period, which is a wider range of scores than is found in inbreds. Average activity scores of inbreds with this dose of cocaine in this apparatus are: 132 ± 16, 119 ± 23, 131 ± 18, 85 ± 27 and 136 ± 17 (Mean ± SEM, N = 6-10) for A, BALB, C3H, C57BL/6 and DBA/2 mice, respectively. In contrast to nicotine, Figure 5 shows that activity scores and body temperature in animals given cocaine are uncorrelated, indicating that for cocaine, the two tests measure different physiological responses to cocaine.

Although we arc in the early stages of these studies, several significant results have already been obtained. The results of the mass screening of HS mice for sensitivity to nicotine and sensitivity to cocaine indicate that a wide range of responses exists within the population for both drugs. The range of responses is greater than that found for any of the common inbred strains we have screened. This indicates that we should be successful in obtaining lines with differential responses to both drugs. Additionally, these data indicate that the HS mice could be extremely useful in studying correlations among multiple behavioral, physiological and biochemical responses to both drugs, as was suggested earlier by McClearn and coworkers.[4] A good example of this is our finding that a strong correlation exists

FIGURE 3. Correlation between Y-maze activity and body temperature following administration of 0.75 mg/kg nicotine in 417 male and female HS mice.

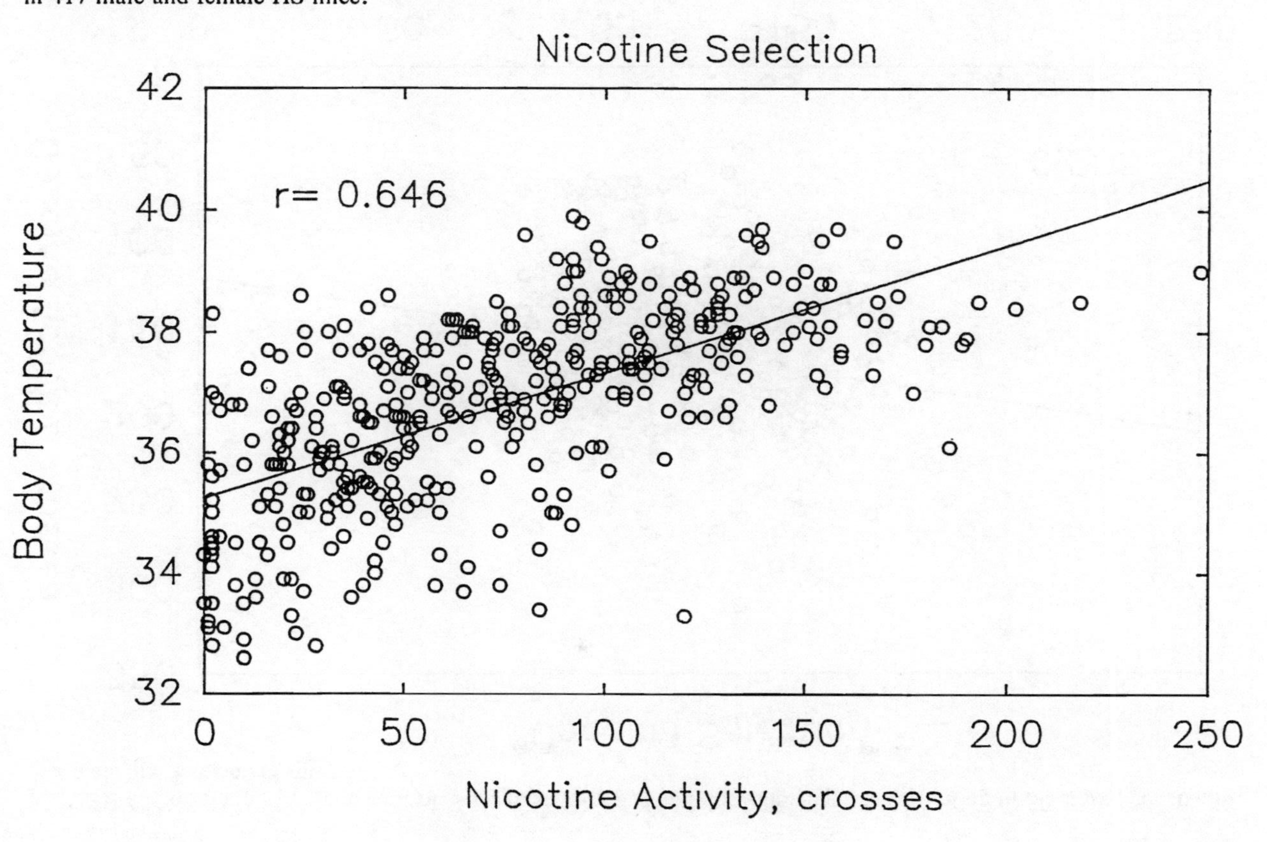

FIGURE 4. Correlation between control Y-maze activity and activity following administration of 50 mg/kg cocaine in 392 male and female HS mice.

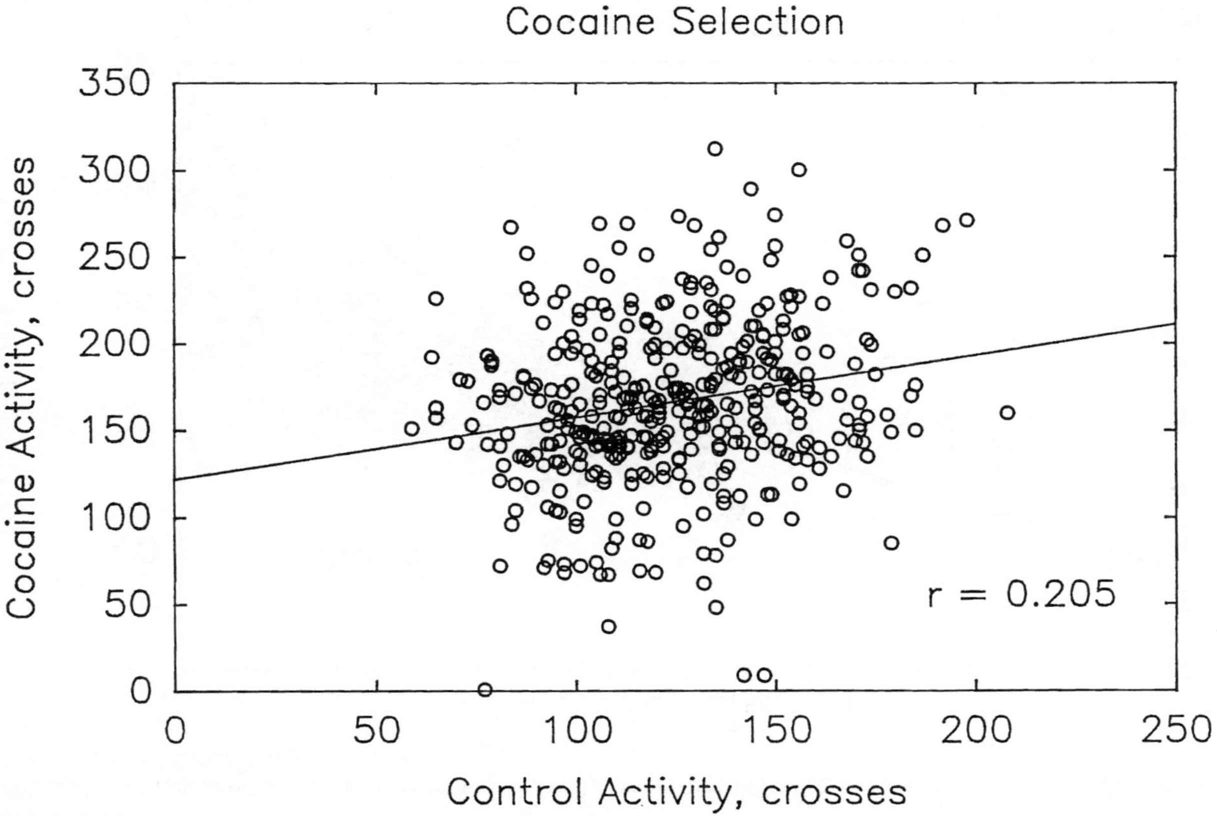

FIGURE 5. Correlation between Y-maze activity and body temperature following administration of 50 mg/kg cocaine in 392 male and female HS mice.

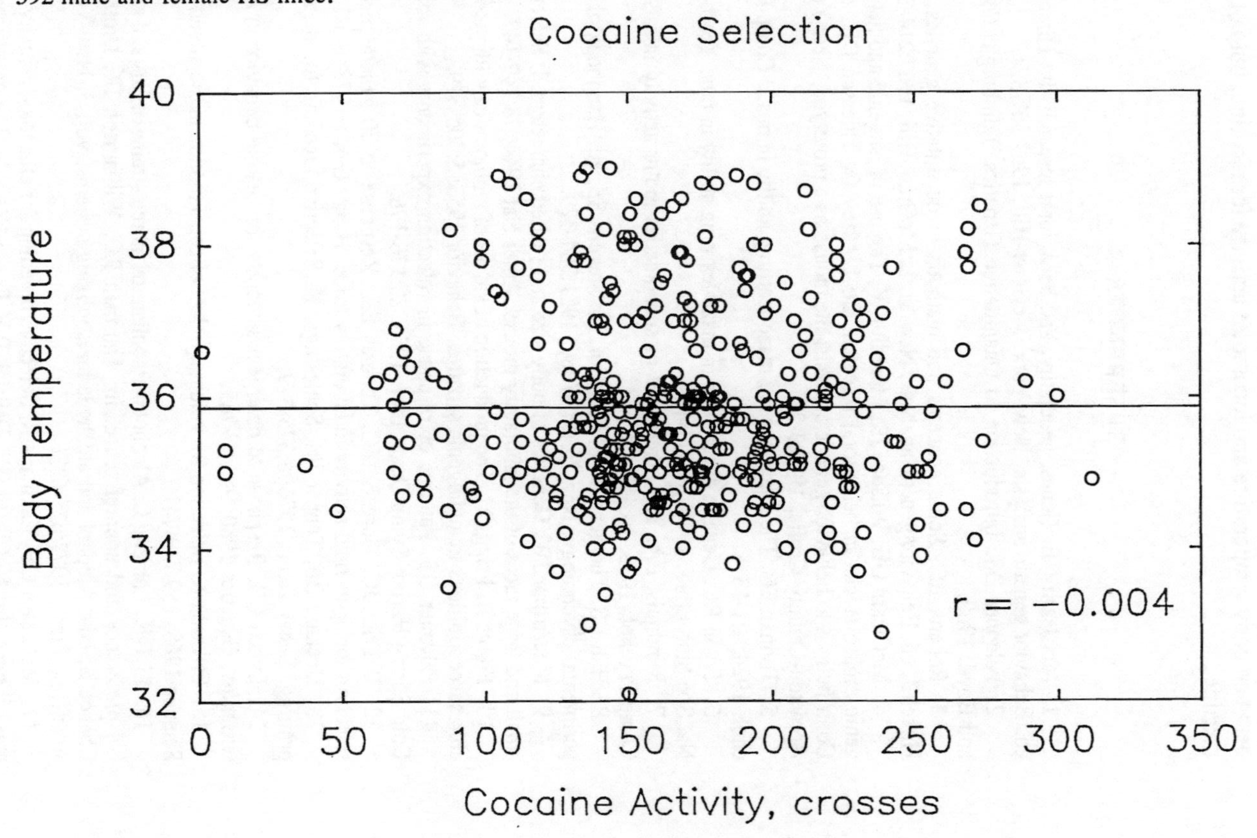

between body temperature and locomotor activity for nicotine, but not for cocaine.

REFERENCES

1. McClearn GE. Genes, generality, and behavioral research. In: Hirsch J, ed. Behavior genetic analysis. New York: McGraw-Hill, 1967:307-321.

2. Falconer DS. Introduction to Quantitative Genetics. Edinburgh: Oliver and Boyd, 1960.

3. Roberts RC. Some concepts and methods in quantitative genetics. In: Hirsch J, ed. Behavior genetic analysis. New York: McGraw-Hill, 1967:214-257.

4. McClearn GE, Wilson, JR, Meredith W. The use of isogenic and heterogenic mouse stocks in behavioral research. In: Lindzey G, Thiessen DD, eds. Contributions to behavior-genetic analysis: the mouse as a prototype, New York: Appleton-Century-Crofts, 1970:3-22.

5. Tolman EC. The inheritance of maze-learning ability in rats. J Comp Psychol. 1924; 4:1-18.

6. Tryon RC. Genetic differences in maze-learning ability in rats. Yearbook Nat Soc Stud Educ. 1940; 39:111-119.

7. Rundquist EA. The inheritance of spontaneous motor activity in rats. J. Comp Psychol. 1933; 16:415-438.

8. Hall CS. The genetics of behavior. In: Stevens SS, ed. Handbook of experimental psychology. New York: Wiley, 1951:304-329.

9. MacArthur JW. Genetics of body size and related characters. I: Selecting small and large races of the laboratory mouse. Amer Nat 1944; 78:142-147.

10. Frings H, Frings M. The production of stocks of albino mice with predictable susceptibilities to audiogenic seizures. Behavior 1953; 5:305-319.

11. Falconer DS. Patterns of response in selection experiments with mice. Cold Spring Harbor Symp Quant Biol. 1955; 20:178-196.

12. DeFries JC, Gervais MC, Thomas EA. Response to 30 generations of selection for open-field activity in laboratory mice. Behav Genet 1978; 8:3-13.

13. Deckard BS, Tepper JM, Schlesinger K. Selective breeding for acoustic priming. Behav Genet 1976; 6:375-379.

14. Lynch CB. Response to divergent selection for nesting behavior in *Mus musculus*. Genetics 1980; 96:757-765.

15. Eriksson K. Selection for voluntary alcohol consumption in the albino rat. Science 1968; 159:739-741.

16. Li T-K, Lumeng L. Alcohol metabolism of inbred strains of rats and alcohol preference and nonpreference. In: Thurman RG, Williamson JR, Drott H, Chance B, eds. Alcohol and aldehyde metabolizing systems, vol. 3. New York: Academic Press, 1977:625-633.

17. McClearn GE, Kakihana R. Selective breeding for ethanol sensitivity: SS and LS mice. In: McClearn GE, Deitrich RA, Erwin VG, eds. The development

of animal models as pharmacogenetic tools. DHHS Publication No. (ADM 81-1133), Washington, D.C.: U.S. Government Printing Office, 1981:147-159.

18. Wilson JR, Erwin VG, DeFries JC, Petersen DR, Cole-Harding S. Ethanol dependence in mice: Direct and correlated responses to ten generations of selective breeding. Behav Genet 1984; 14:235-256.

19. Crabbe JC, Kosobud A, Young ER, Tam BR, McSwigan JD. Bidirectional selection for susceptibility to ethanol withdrawal seizures in *Mus musculus*. Behav Genet 1985; 15:521-536.

20. Crabbe JC, Kosobud A, Tam BR, Young ER, Deutsch CM. Genetic selection of mouse lines sensitive (COLD) and resistant (HOT) to acute ethanol hypothermia. Alcohol Drug Res 1987; 7:163-174.

21. Crabbe JC, Young ER, Deutsch CM, Tam BR, Kosobud A. Mice genetically selected for differences in open-field activity after ethanol. Pharmacol Biochem Behav 1987; 27:577-581.

22. Gallaher EJ, Gionet SE. Initial sensitivity and tolerance to ethanol in mice genetically selected for diazepam sensitivity Alcoholism: Clin Exp Res 1988; 12:77-80.

23. Belkanp JK, Danielson PW, Laursen SE, Noordewier B. Selective breeding for levorphanol-induced antinociception on the hot-plate assay: commonalties in mechanism of action with morphine, petazocine, ethylketoclazocine, U-50488H and clonidine in mice. J Pharmacol Exp Ther 1987; 241:477-481.

24. DeFries JC. Selective breeding for behavioral and pharmacological responses in laboratory mice. In: Gershon E, Matthysse SI, Breakefield XO, Ciaranello RO, eds. Basic research strategies for psychobiology and psychiatry. The Boxwood Press: New York, 1981:199-214.

25. DeFries JC. Current perspectives on selective breeding: Example and theory. In: McClearn GE, Deitrich RA, Erwin VG, eds. The development of animal models as pharmacogenetic tools. DHHS Publication No. (ADM 81-1133), Washington, D.C.: U.S. Government Printing Office, 1981:11-35.

26. Lynch CB. Report on the task group on design of selection experiments. In: McClearn GE, Deitrich RA, Erwin VG, eds. The development of animal models as pharmacogenetic tools. DHHS Publication No. (ADM 81-1133), Washington, D.C.: U.S. Government Printing Office, 1981:269-275.

27. Roberts RC. Current perspectives on selective breeding: Theoretical aspects. In: McClearn GE, Deitrich RA, Erwin VG, eds. The Development of animal models as pharmacogenetic tools. DHHS Publication No. (ADM 81-1133), Washington, D.C.: U.S. Government Printing Office, 1981:37-58.

28. Henderson ND. Interpreting studies which compare high- and low-selected lines. Behav Genet 1989; 19:473-502.

29. Henningfield JE, Miyasato K, Jasinski DR. Cigarette smokers self-administer intravenous nicotine. Pharmacol Biochem Behav 1983; 19:887-890.

30. Nagoshi CT, Wilson JR, Plomin R. Use of regression residuals to quantify individual differences in acute sensitivity and tolerance to ethanol. Alcoholism: Clin Exp Res 1986; 10:343-349.

31. Cohen J, Cohen P. Applied multiple regression/correlation analysis for the behavioral sciences. Hillsdale, NJ: Lawrence Erlbaum Associates, 1983.
32. Crabbe JC, Weigle RM. Quantification of individual sensitivities to ethanol in selective breeding experiments: Difference scores versus regression residuals. Alcoholism: Clin Exp Res 1987; 11:544-549.

Where Are the mu Receptors That Mediate Opioid Analgesia? An Autoradiographic Study in the HAR and LAR Selection Lines

J. K. Belknap, PhD
S. E. Laursen, BS
K. E. Sampson, BS
A. Wilkie, BS

SUMMARY. One line (strain) of mouse has been selectively bred in our laboratory for 15 generations to exhibit a very high sensitivity to levorphanol-induced analgesia on the hot plate assay (HAR or high antinociceptive response line). Concurrently, a second line (LAR or low antinociceptive response line) has been bred in the opposite direction, i.e., to exhibit a very low sensitivity under the same conditions. This has resulted in a 7-fold difference in sensitivity between HAR and LAR mice as a result of changes in gene frequency. Receptor autoradiographic studies with 3H-DAGO were carried out in the central gray to find receptor populations differing greatly in density between HAR and LAR mice to parallel their *in vivo* sensitivity differences: such receptors would then be implicated in mediating *in vivo* analgesia. The caudal portions of the dorsal raphe nucleus (DRN) showed 1.5- to 2-fold differences in density of

J. K. Belknap is affiliated with the Research Service (151W), VA Medical Center, and Department of Medical Psychology, Oregon Health Sciences University, Portland, OR 97201 and Departments of Pharmacology and Neuroscience, University of North Dakota, Grand Forks, ND 58202. S. E. Laursen, K. E. Sampson and A. Wilkie are affiliated with the Departments of Pharmacology and Neuroscience, University of North Dakota, Grand Forks, ND 58202.

This work was supported by NIDA Grants DA05228, DA02723, NIDA Contract No. 271-87-8120 and a VA Merit Review Grant. Appreciation is extended to Dr. Miles Herkenham for allowing the author to learn receptor autoradiography in his laboratory, and for helpful comments on an earlier version of the manuscript.

mu sites, while the periaqueductal gray (PAG) showed relatively small differences. These results strongly suggest that mu receptors in a portion of the DRN are involved in mediating analgesia due to systemically administered opioids in this population of mice.

INTRODUCTION

Selective breeding refers to a system of mating where only those individuals possessing a desired characteristic are allowed to breed, and thus contribute genes to subsequent generations.[1] This procedure has been practiced since time of the ancients, and its success is reflected in the hundreds of widely differing breeds of dogs, cattle and other domesticated species fashioned by animal breeders. The remarkable differences that exist between breeds of dogs, for example, attests to the tremendous power of selective breeding in producing organisms tailor-made for a specific purpose. In spite of its long history in agricultural and livestock breeding, selective breeding as a tool in scientific research is of much more recent origin.

The purpose of selective breeding (selection) in modern research is generally as follows: (1) to perform certain types of quantitative genetic analyses, such as the assessment of heritability and of shared genetic determination with other traits (correlated responses), (2) to breed organisms with desirable characteristics for research, and (3) to use the selection lines as an hypothesis testing tool concerning the mechanisms, determinants, effects and correlates of the trait under selection.[1] Many examples of the usefulness of this approach with regard to drugs of abuse can be found in recent reviews,[1-4] and in the contributions by Froehlich, Gallaher and Smolen from this meeting.

With regard to opioids, only three selection projects prior to the present one have been described in the literature. Nichols and Hsiao[5] selectively bred rats for high and for low consumption of (and preference for) morphine after the animals had previously been serially injected with morphine and subsequently withdrawn. This selection project was successful in that a large divergence between the two oppositely-selected lines (about 4-fold) was achieved in voluntary morphine consumption in only the third generation of selective breeding. Judson and Goldstein[6] bidirectionally selected for both high and low levorphanol-induced locomotor activity (running fit) in mice. After three generations of selection, a 3.5-fold difference between the high (runner) and low (nonrunner) selection lines was evident. Selection progress was unusually rapid in the low activity line, suggesting that there may be one or two genes accounting for this rapid response.[6] Panocka et al.[7] selectively bred for cold water swim (stress)-induced analgesia in both directions in the HA (high analgesia) and LA (low analgesia) lines, respectively, using the hot plate assay. This type of analgesia was naloxone sensitive (1.0 mg/kg) in HA mice, but not in LA mice, implying mediation by endogenous opioids in the HA mice.[8] These two lines also differed markedly in their analgesic sensitivity to morphine on the hot plate assay, suggesting extensive commonalities in mechanisms between cold water- and morphine-induced analgesia.

THE HAR AND LAR SELECTION LINES

Beginning with a genetically outbred stock (Binghamton HET), 15 generations of selective breeding have been carried out in our laboratories for high (HAR) and for low (LAR) sensitivity to i.p. levorphanol on the hot plate assay. The initial development and progress of selective breeding up to generation 4 has been previously described.[9] Since the 5th generation, all first litter mice in each generation (N = 190-310) were hot plate tested with and without i.p. levorphanol, and the highest scoring 25%-30% of the HAR line, and the lowest scoring 25%-30% of the LAR line, were selected to serve as breeders for the next generation of the HAR and LAR selection lines, respectively. The hot plate testing procedure has been previously described.[9,10] The index used to select breeders was the ratio of hot plate latencies following i.p. levorphanol to the latencies seen without drug administration, assessed two days later. The dose of levorphanol used was that which doubled no drug latencies in the immediately prior generation of each line.[11] This insured roughly equivalent hot plate latencies in both HAR and LAR lines (about 18-24 sec), but the dose necessary to accomplish this was 5 to 7-fold higher in the LAR line compared to the HAR line in the later generations (see below). Both lines were maintained by 12-16 successful breeding pairs per generation. Mass selection was used in each generation through generation 10 for the reasons previously given,[9] and within family (within litter) selection used thereafter to retard inbreeding once selection progress had reached an apparent plateau.

The results of the first 15 generations of selective breeding are shown in Figure 1 in terms of the percent of maximum possible effect (%MPE). Selection progress in the high (HAR) and low (LAR) directions was somewhat asymmetrical, which is not uncommon in the selective breeding literature.[12] In the high line (HAR), selection progress was relatively rapid, reaching its maximal extent at about generation 4, with little selection

FIGURE 1. The progress in selective breeding over 15 generations for high (HAR) and for low (LAR) sensitivity to levorphanol-induced analgesia in terms of the degree of analgesia (%MPE) per unit dose (1 mg/kg) of levorphanol tartrate on the plate assay (52.5°C). The standard errors are not shown, since half of them are smaller than the symbols used to denote the generation means (N = 61 to 140 per point). The hot plate test was administered only once 20 min following an i.p. injection of levorphanol. The behavioral end point was hind paw lift, lick or shake, whichever occurred first.[9,10] Hot plate latency scores (sec) were converted to percent of maximum possible effect (%MPE) by the formula: %MPE = [latency(drug) - latency(no drug)] × 100 / [90 - latency(no drug)].

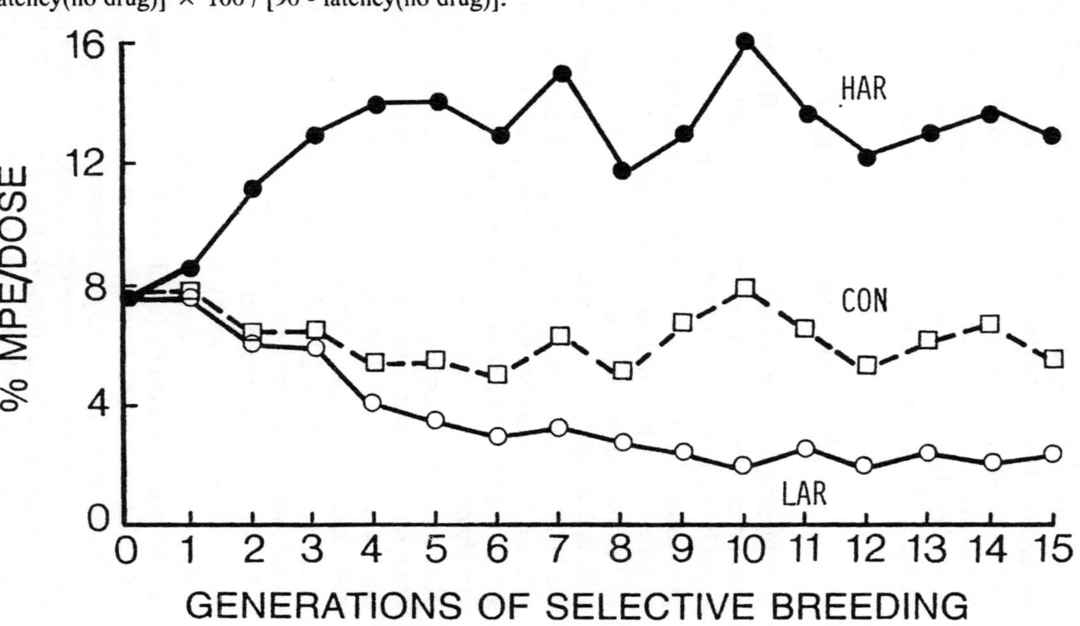

progress evident thereafter despite continued selective breeding. This is suggestive of a relatively few genes having a major impact on enhanced sensitivity to levorphanol, which became fixed relatively rapidly in the high line. In contrast, progress in the low direction (LAR) was slower and more gradual, reaching its maximal extent at about the 10th generation (see Figure 1), suggesting a relatively larger number of genes, each with relatively small effects on diminished sensitivity to levorphanol.[12] The fluctuations affecting all three lines from generation to generation in Figure 1 are probably due to environmental factors such as a move to a new animal facility (generation 2), a complete change in technical staff performing the hot plate testing (generations 8 and 11), and a change in testing room (generation 12). Since selection progress had reached an asymptote, further selective breeding was suspended beginning at generation 16, except for the application of selection pressure to eliminate the small differences seen in the absence of drug administration. Despite this, the difference between the lines in generation 18 and 19, when the present autoradiographic work was done, remains almost the same as at generation 10 or 15.

Figure 2 shows a dose-response curve for levorphanol in HAR, LAR and CON (nonselected control) mice of the 10th generation. The difference between the HAR and LAR lines seen with levorphanol was similar to that seen with morphine (7.0-fold vs. 8.6-fold in the slopes of the dose-response curves), indicating that the genes which determine the levorphanol response are largely the same genes operating with morphine,[11] as would be expected given their similar pharmacology. In contrast to the large differences in analgesia induced by i.p. levorphanol or morphine, these two lines differed only slightly with saline injections (2 sec).[11] In the most recent generation (22nd), they do not differ at all on the hot plate with either saline injections or no injections (unpublished).

These lines do not differ appreciably in brain levorphanol or morphine concentrations at the time of hot plate testing when given equal doses of either drug,[11] indicating that the two lines do not differ importantly in drug disposition or metabolism. Other studies in our laboratory have shown that the differences between the lines in levorphanol-induced analgesia are even greater with the i.c.v. route compared to the i.p. route of administration.[13] Among a series of opioid analgesics, HAR vs. LAR differences were greatest with predominantly mu agonists such as morphine, levorphanol and DAGO, and were smallest with predominantly kappa or delta agonists, such as U50488H, DSLET and DPDPE,[11,14] indicating that

FIGURE 2. Dose-response curve for i.p. levorphanol in LAR, HAR and CON (control) mice from generation 10 on the hot plate assay. Results for later generations are similar. Hot plate scores are in terms of latencies (sec) to respond with a hind paw lift, lick or shake, whichever occurred first (all involve a paw lift). A dose rather than log dose plot is used because the former yields a better linear fit (all r's > .97). Despite the large differences in latencies between HAR and LAR mice when given levorphanol, only a small difference (2 sec) was seen following saline injections. Each point represents the mean of 10-24 mice. The regression (b) values are also shown for each line.

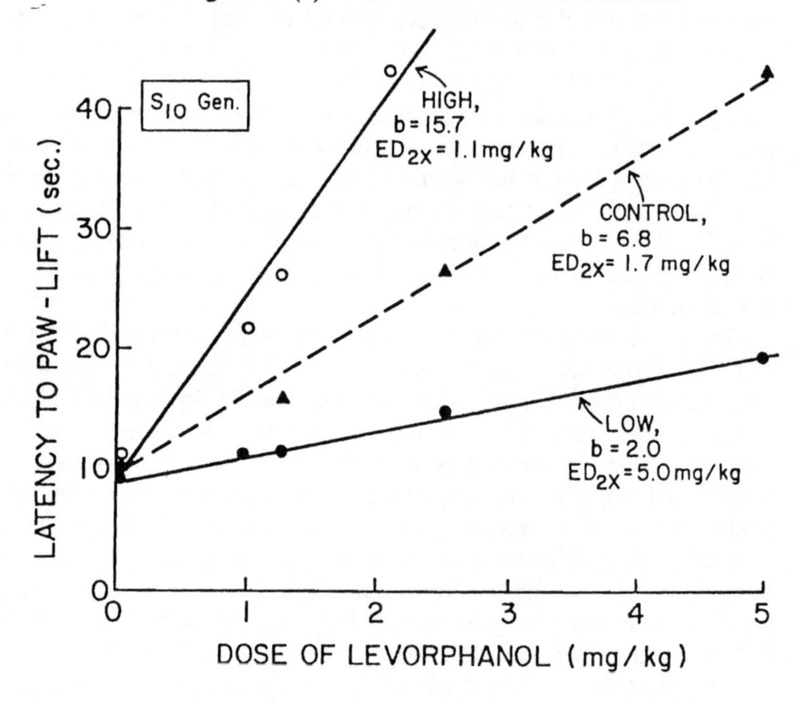

selective breeding has primarily altered the function of mu receptors relative to the other two subtypes. In the present studies, we utilized this genetic animal model to determine which populations of mu opioid receptors *in vitro* mediate analgesia *in vivo* through the use of receptor autoradiography. Our working hypothesis assumed that those receptors mediating analgesia would probably show large differences in density between the HAR and LAR lines as a result of selective breeding, assuming an appreciable heritability. In contrast, those receptors irrelevant to analgesia probably would show no differences.

MU OPIOID RECEPTOR AUTORADIOGRAPHY

The technique for preparation and sectioning of the brain is patterned after that of Herkenham and Pert.[15] Following decapitation, each brain was carefully dissected free on an ice-cold plate. The excised brain was frozen by immersion in isopentane at −20° C for 60 seconds. Twenty micron sections were made at cryostat temperatures of −14 to −18° C and thaw-mounted onto pre-cooled gelatin-coated (subbed) slides. Sections were then dried overnight at 4° C in a desiccator jar with desiccant. Each HAR mouse brain was processed together with a LAR mouse brain as a matched pair, and run through the entire procedure concurrently, including incubation in the same bath and development on the same sheet of tritium sensitive film (see below). Subsequent data analysis was based on differences between matched pairs to maximize comparability between the lines.

The slides were preincubated for 20 min in ice cold 170 mM Tris, pH 7.4, and incubated for 60 minutes in the same buffer containing 3.3 nM 3H-DAGO (NEN, 35 Ci/mmol), followed by three washes in ice cold buffer for 20 sec each, and a final "in and out" dip in distilled water to remove salts. Because nonspecific binding was quite low (average of 8%), total binding was used in all subsequent analyses. The slides were dried within 90 sec with a hair dryer at a low heat setting and allowed to stand overnight. The slides were then exposed for five weeks to tritium sensitive film (Hyperfilm, Amersham) by direct contact in an X-ray cassette at room temperature.

Commercially available tritium standards for autoradiography (Tritium Microscales, Amersham) were used to convert optical density to nCi/mg tissue. These standards were constructed based on nCi per mg of rat brain gray matter,[15] and thus are only approximate for mouse brain. An important problem for quantitative work is the quenching of tritium by brain lipids, causing underestimates of up to 30% of true 3H-ligand concentrations in rat brain gray matter.[16-19] The standards are designed to correct for quenching in gray matter, but this correction may not be entirely appropriate for mouse brain compared to rat brain. This is less problematic in the present study, since we are comparing the same anatomical area from two different brains (HAR vs. LAR), where the degree of quenching is presumably similar in the two selectively-bred lines.

These receptor autoradiographic studies focused on the midbrain PAG, since this structure has been widely implicated as an important site of analgesic action. 3H-DAGO was selected because it is among the most mu selective ligands presently available, and there is much evidence implicating the mu opioid receptor as the most important subtype for morphine analgesia,[20] especially that associated with a thermal stimulus.[21] The first series of slides (Series 1) was taken at intervals along most of the length of the PAG in four matched pairs of HAR and LAR mice. Coronal sections were taken corresponding to those numbered 351, 397, 423 and 437 as shown in the atlas of Sidman et al.,[21] or −3.2, −4.2, −4.8 and −5.4 mm caudal to Bregma as shown in the atlas of Slotnik and Leonard.[23] These sections ranged through about a 2.2 mm length of the PAG. Because apparent selection line differences were seen in this series at the level of the dorsal raphe nucleus (DRN), which was most marked at sections 423 and 437, a second series of sections (Series 2) was taken in ten matched pairs of mice from sections 397 through 455 (1.5 mm length) at 40 micron intervals. This series encompassed the area of highest 3H-DAGO binding in the DRN, and the only portion where differences between the lines were evident.

Average binding densities in the DRN and surrounding PAG were determined by microcomputer image analysis (MicroComp DS System, So. Micro Instr., Atlanta, GA). Our initial autoradiographic studies (Series 1) found that there were small but significant differences (two-tailed t test) between HAR and LAR mice in mu receptor binding along most of the length of the PAG. Mean (± SD) 3H-DAGO binding in the PAG was 1.06 ± 0.11 nCi/mg in the HAR mice and 0.91 ± 0.11 nCi/mg in the LAR mice (4 mice per line, 4 sections per mouse = 16 determinations per line). Binding densities were fairly uniform from the rostral to caudal sections of both lines. Binding was higher in the lateral aspects of the PAG, especially in the dorsolateral portions in the more rostral sections, and in the ventrolateral portions of the more caudal sections in both lines. However, much larger differences (about 2-fold) were found in mu receptor binding in the DRN, but only at the sections corresponding to those numbered 423 and 437, in the more caudal portions of the DRN. For these sections, the mean (± SD) density values were 2.4 ± 0.5 (HAR) and 1.3 ± 0.5 (LAR) nCi/mg and the peak density values were 5.6 ± 1.1 (HAR) vs. 2.5 ± 0.7 (LAR), means ± SD, N = 8 determinations per line, $p < .01$). This was confirmed in Series 2, where the area of maximum DRN binding, which was also the area where the differences between the lines were most evident, was at sections numbered 431 to 437 from the Sidman et al.[22] mouse atlas (about −5.0 to −5.3 mm caudal to Bregma), in the more caudal portions of the DRN. This area of maximum binding appears as a visually distinct "hot spot" just below the floor of the aqueduct in the HAR autoradiographs (Figure 3), and was quite small,

FIGURE 3. Receptor autoradiograph of a coronal section from a HAR mouse at about -5.0 mm caudal to Bregma. The arrow points to the area of high binding in a portion of the DRN just below the floor of the aquaduct. In contrast, this same area taken from LAR mice is only slightly more dense than the surrounding PAG (not shown) . The autoradiograph was labelled with 3.3 nM 3H-DAGO on tritium sensitive film (Amersham Ultrofilm) as described in Methods, and is representative of the HAR mice studied.

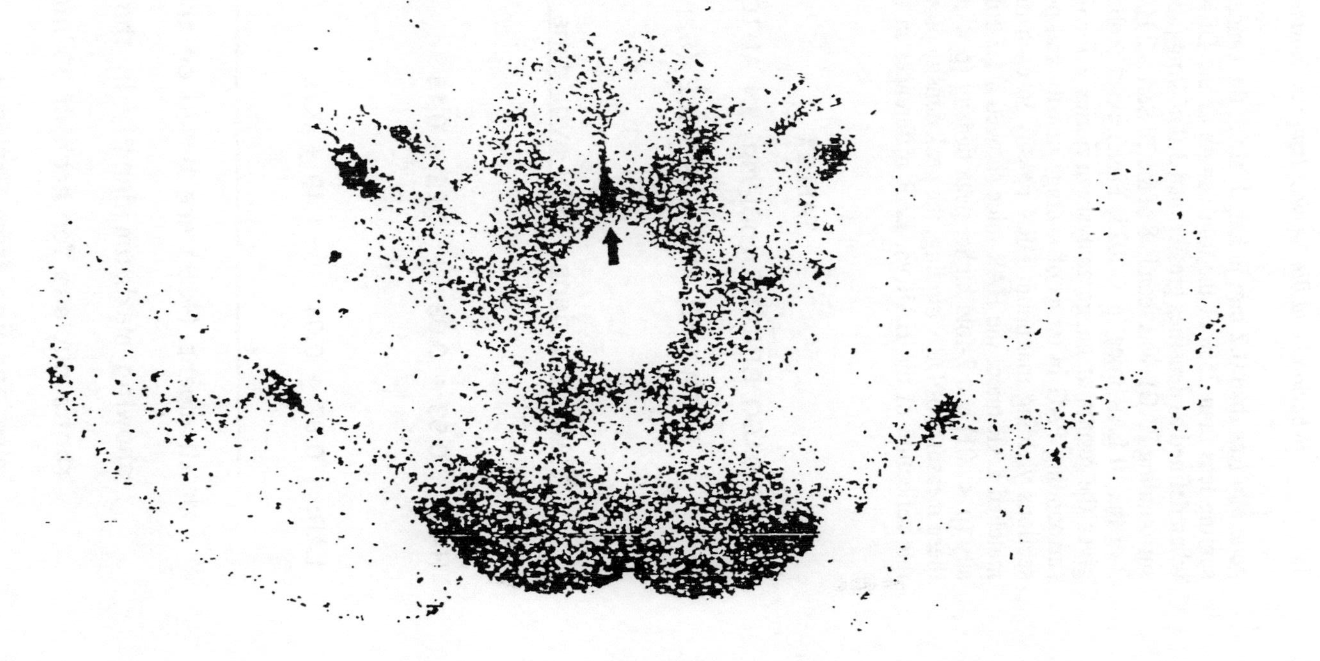

generally less than 0.2 mm in length along the caudal/rostral axis, representing less than 25% of the total length of the DRN. This "hot spot," when defined as densities greater than 3.0 nCi/mg (about 3-fold above the surrounding PAG), was seen in 8 of the 10 Series 2 HAR mice, but in only 2 of the 10 LAR mice ($p < .025$, Fisher exact probability test). Table 1 gives the results of image analysis in Series 2 for the caudal DRN and surrounding PAG in terms of average density and peak density at those sections yielding maximum DRN density in each mouse. Compared to matched LAR mice, the HAR mice showed a 1.5-fold higher mean density ($p < .01$) and 2-fold higher peak density ($p < .01$) in the DRN. Of these measures of DRN binding, the peak density provides the most accurate reflection of the HAR vs. LAR differences in the "hot spot" area

TABLE 1

3H-DAGO BINDING (nCi/mg) IN AUTORADIOGRAPHS

FROM HAR AND LAR MICE (Series 2)

	PAG avg. dens.	DRN avg. dens.	DRN peak
HAR:	0.93 ± 0.03	2.22 ± 0.18	4.8 ± 0.5
LAR:	0.87 ± 0.04	1.49 ± 0.19	2.6 ± 0.4

* All means (±SE) are based on the sections showing maximum density in the dorsal raphe nucleus for each of 10 individual mice per line from Series 2.

than does the mean DRN density, because the latter encompassed all of the DRN visible in the coronal sections, while the "hot spot" was found only in the most dorsal portions of the DRN closest to the aqueduct. In contrast to these marked differences in the DRN, no significant differences were seen in the surrounding PAG measured on the same autoradiographs, although there was a trend in the expected direction ($p < .3$, Series 2, two-tailed t test).

CONCLUSIONS

Selective breeding has effectively altered gene frequencies for those genes which influence hot plate-assessed analgesia, resulting in two lines of mice which differ markedly in their genetically-based sensitivity to opioid-induced analgesia on the hot plate assay. By generation 10, the apparent limits of selection had been attained. This rapid progress is largely due to the rather high degree of genetic control of this trait (heritability of 32%),[9] and the use of mass selection, which is usually maximally efficient and effective compared to other systems of mating.[9,12]

As selective breeding causes changes in gene frequency affecting analgesia, parallel changes should also occur in those receptors responsible for analgesia, assuming they are heritable to an appreciable extent. In contrast, no changes would be expected for receptors irrelevant to analgesia within the limits of sampling error (e.g., genetic drift). Only small differences (16%) were found between HAR and LAR mice in mu receptor density along most the length of the PAG in Series 1, and no significant differences were found in Series 2, although the trend was in the same direction. Series 1 encompassed most of the length of the PAG, whereas Series 2 involved only that portion of the PAG where DRN binding was greatest, generally in the more caudal sections. It should be noted that selective breeding can only alter receptor populations to the degree that they are heritable.[12] Thus, it is possible that mu receptor densities in the PAG were not greatly changed by selective breeding because of a low heritability compared to those in the DRN. In contrast to these small and somewhat equivocal PAG differences, consistent and much larger differences were found in mu receptor binding in the dorsal and caudal portions of the DRN, where 1.5 to 2-fold differences were found. Thus, mu receptors in a small portion of the DRN appear to be one site mediating the analgesic effects of systematically administered levorphanol or morphine in HAR/LAR mice. It is likely that other receptor sites will be found as this approach is extended to other areas, such as the restroventral medulla and the spinal cord.

Previous studies in our laboratory using whole brain or spinal cord homogenates have found only small (< 25%) or no differences between HAR and LAR mice in Bmax and K_D values for tritiated naloxone, dihydromorphine or DSLET binding.[23] More recent studies in our laboratory (unpublished) also found small or no differences in homogenates from midbrain, hypothalamus, cortex and medulla with these same ligands. Whole brain homogenate studies with 3H-DAGO showed very small (< 10%) or no differences for any binding parameter in mice taken from the same generation as the autoradiographic data (unpublished). Since the opioid receptors mediating analgesia appear to represent only a small proportion of the total number of opioid receptors, this type of "grind and bind" study does not appear to have the resolving power to discriminate those receptors relevant to analgesia from the much larger number that are not. The present autoradiographic data suggest that the relevant receptors mediating hot plate-assessed analgesia do indeed represent a very small proportion of the total number of mu sites in the midbrain, and moreover, they are probably located in narrowly circumscribed areas. The present findings suggest that studies into the mechanisms of analgesic action of opioids (e.g., second messenger systems, ion channels), should include the DRN since it is highly likely to be a fruitful area compared to whole brain or crude midbrain preparations. Furthermore, the difficulty in showing receptor changes due to chronic tolerance development may be due to the inability of brain homogenate studies to detect the highly localized changes that may underly tolerance.

While the site(s) of analgesic action of morphine and similar opioids is not precisely known, most recent microinjection and electrophysiological studies suggest three sites as being most likely: the midbrain periaqueductal gray (PAG), rostroventral medulla (n. raphe magnus, n. reticularis gigantocellularis, n. reticularis paragigantocellularis) and the dorsal horn of the spinal cord (especially laminae I and II).[25-28] Microinjection of morphine can produce marked analgesia at all three sites, as does electrical brain stimulation via microelectrodes.[28,29] The ventrolateral PAG is more sensitive to microinjected morphine than other portions of the PAG.[28,30] Closely associated with the ventromedial PAG is the dorsal raphe nucleus (DRN), a structure that is sensitive to microinjected morphine, although apparently less so than the ventrolateral PAG.[30] However, the DRN has received comparatively little attention as a site mediating opioid analgesia compared to the PAG or the nucleus raphe magnus (NRM) in the rostroventral medulla.

Of all the evidence in the literature concerning the site(s) of action for systemically administered opioids, microinjection and electrical stimulation studies have had the greatest impact on our present thinking. A key assumption in such studies is that the sites most sensitive to microinjected morphine or electrical stimulation are most likely to be the ones active when opioids are systemically administered. While a very plausible assumption, there may be exceptions, whereby critical sites mediating analgesia with systemic administration may not be among the most sensitive sites to these localized treatments. A possible example of this is the DRN, which is apparently not the most sensitive site to microinjection in the central gray, but is implicated as a site mediating analgesia in the present report. Moreover, the synergistic (multiplicative) interaction between two or more sites may be of critical importance with systemic administration, as appears to be the case between spinal cord and supraspinal sites.[31,32] When synergism between two or more sites is important, the sensitivity to microinjected morphine or electrical stimulation at only one site will likely lead to an underestimation of its importance under systemic administration. However, detecting such interactions, whether synergistic or inhibitory, would be a formidable task because of the many-fold increase in effort needed to assess sites in combination compared to the usual cases, where only one site at a time is studied. In addition, there are the well-known problems with local drug administration and electrical stimulation that make extrapolation to systemic administration difficult, such as effects due to diffusion to other sites away from the site of application, and nonspecific effects due to locally high concentrations of the drug or electrical current at the site of application.[32] A major advantage of the genetic/autoradiographic approach employed in this report is that it circumvents all of the disadvantages noted above. However, a major disadvantage is that receptor populations must be heritable to an appreciable extent (i.e., some proportion of the observed variability must be genetically determined) for differences between oppositely selected lines to materialize. Fortunately, in the selective breeding literature, only a small proportion of traits subjected to or associated with selective breeding have been found to be insufficiently heritable.[12] However, the heritability of anatomically discrete receptor populations is essentially uncharted territory, so unequivocal conclusions cannot be drawn. A second disadvantage is that selectively-bred lines must exist for the trait of interest, and at present, the HAR and LAR lines are the only ones available involving administered opioids. On balance, the strengths and weaknesses of the genetic autoradiographic approach nicely complement those of other approaches, and thus the former has potentially much to add to our knowledge gained from other sources.

REFERENCES

1. Crabbe, J.C., Phillips, T.J., Kosobud, A. and Belknap, J.K. Estimation of genetic correlation: Interpretation of experiments using selectively bred and inbred animals. Alcoholism: Clin. Exp. Res., in press.

2. Frischknecht, H.R., Siegfried, B. and Waser, P.G., Opioids and behavior: Genetic aspects. Experientia 44:473-481, 1988.

3. Phillips, T.J., Crabbe, J.C. and Feller, D.J. Selected mouse lines, alcohol, and behavior. Experientia 45:805-827, 1989.

4. Belknap, J.K. and O'Toole, L.A. Studies of genetic differences in response to opioid drugs. In Harris, R.A. and Crabbe, J.C. (Eds.) The Genetic Basis of Alcohol and Drug Actions, Plenum, NY, NY, in press.

5. Nichols, J.R. and Hsiao, S. Addiction liability of albino rats: Breeding for quantitative differences in morphine drinking. Science 157:561-563, 1967.

6. Judson, B.A. and Goldstein, A. Genetic control of opiate-induced locomotor activity in mice. J. Pharmacol. Exp. Ther. 206:56-60, 1978.

7. Panocka, I., Marek, P. and Sadowski, B. Inheritance of stress-induced analgesia in mice. Selective breeding study. Brain Res. 397:152-155, 1986.

8. Panocka, I., Marek, P. and Sadowski, B. Differentiation of neurochemical basis of stress-induced analgesia in mice by selective breeding. Brain Res. 397:156-160, 1986.

9. Belknap, J.K., Haltli, N.R., Goebel, D.M. and Lamé, M. Selective breeding for high and for low levels of opiate-induced analgesia in mice. Behavior Genetics 13:383-395, 1983.

10. Belknap, J.K., Lamé, M. and Danielson, P.W. Inbred strain differences in morphine-induced analgesia with the hot plate assay: A reassessment. Behavior Genetics, 20: (in press).

11. Belknap, J.K., Danielson, P.W., Laursen, S.E. and Noordewier, B. Selective breeding for levorphanol-induced antinociception on the hot plate assay: Commonalities in mechanisms of action with morphine, pentazocine, ethylketocyclazocine, U-50488H and clonidine in mice. J. Pharmacol. Exp. Ther., 241:477-481, 1987.

12. Falconer, D.S. An Introduction to Quantitative Genetics, Longmans, NY, NY, 1981.

13. Laursen, S.E. and Belknap, J.K. Intracerebroventricular (i.c.v.) injections in mice: Some methodological refinements. J. Pharmacol. Methods 16:355-357, 1986.

14. Belknap, J.K. and Laursen, S.E. DSLET (D-Ser^2-Leu^5 enkephalin-Thr^6) produces analgesia on the hot plate by mechanisms largely different from DAGO and morphine-like opioids. Life Sciences, 41:391-395, 1987.

15. Herkenham, M. and Pert, C.B. Light microscopic localization of brain

opiate receptors: A general autoradiographic method which preserves tissue quality. J. Neurosci. 2:1129-1149, 1982.

16. Geary, W.A., Toga, A.W. and Wooten, G.F. Quantitative film autoradiography for tritium: Methodological considerations. Brain Res. 337:99-108, 1985.

17. Rainbow, T.C., Biegon, A. and Berck, D.J. Quantitative receptor autoradiography with tritium-labeled ligands: Comparison of biochemical and densitometric measurements. J. Neurosci. Methods 11:231-241, 1984.

18. Herkenham, M. Levels of quantitative analysis of receptor autoradiography: Technical and Theoretical Issues. In Brown, R.M., Friedman, D.P. and Nimit, Y. Neuroscience Methods in Drug Abuse Research, NIDA Res. Monogr. No. 62, USGPO, Washington, DC, 1985, pp. 13-29.

19. Herkenham, M. Receptor autoradiography: Optimizing anatomical resolution. In Leslie, F. and Altar, C. (Ed.) Receptor Localization, Part A: Ligand Autoradiography, Alan R. Liss, NY, NY, 1988.

20. Pasternak, G.W. Multiple morphine and enkephalin receptors and the relief of pain. J.A.M.A. 259:1362-1367, 1988.

21. Tyers, M.B. A classification of opiate receptors that mediate antinociception in animals. Br. J. Pharmacol. 69:503-512, 1980.

22. Sidman, R.L., Angevine, J.B. and Pierce, E.T. Atlas of the Mouse Brain and Spinal Cord, Harvard Univ. Press, 1971.

23. Slotnik, B. and Leonard, C.M. A. Stereotaxic Atlas of the Albino Mouse Forebrain. USDHEW-PHS, USGPO, Washington, DC, 1975.

24. Belknap, J.K., Danielson, P.W. and Laursen, S.E. *In vitro* binding to mu and delta opioid receptors as predictors of *in vivo* levorphanol-induced antinociception. Federation Proceedings 44:567, 1985.

25. Gebhart, G.F. Opiate and opioid peptide effects on brain stem neurons: Relevance to nociception and antinociceptive mechanisms. Pain 12:93-140, 1982.

26. Gebhart, G.F. Recent developments in the neurochemical bases of pain and analgesia. In Brown, R.M. et al., (Eds.) Contemporary Research in Pain and Analgesia, 1983, NIDA Res. Monogr. No. 45, USGPO, Washington, DC, 1983.

27. Fields, H.F. Recent advances in research on pain and analgesia. In Brown, R.M. et al., (Eds.) Contemporary Research in Pain and Analgesia, 1983, NIDA Res. Monogr. No. 45, USGPO, Washington, DC, 1983.

28. Fields, H.F. Brainstem mechanisms of pain modulation. In Kruger, L. and Liebeskind, J.C. (Eds.) Advances in Pain Research and Therapy, Vol. 6. Raven Press, NY, NY, 1984.

29. Bodnar, R.J., Williams, C.L., Lee, S.J. and Pasternak, G.W. Role of mu-1 opiate receptors in supraspinal opiate analgesia: a microinjection study. Brain Res. 447:25-34, 1988.

30. Yaksh, T.L. Central nervous system sites mediating opiate analgesia. In Bonica, J.J. (Ed.) Advances in Pain Research and Therapy, Raven Press, NY, NY, pp. 411-426, 1979.

31. Yeung, J.C. and Rudy, T.A. Multiplicative interaction between narcotic agonisms expressed at spinal and supraspinal sites of antinociceptive action as

revealed by concurrent intrathecal and intracerebroventricular injections of morphine. J. Pharmacol. Exp. Ther. 215:633-642, 1980.

32. Yaksh, T.L. Opioid receptors systems and the endorphins: A review of their spinal organization. J. Neurosurg. 67:157-176, 1987.

33. Myers, R.D. Handbook of Drug and Chemical Stimulation of the Brain. Van Nostrand Reinhold, NY, NY, 1974.

Behavioral and Neurochemical Studies in Diazepam-Sensitive and -Resistant Mice

Edward J. Gallaher, PhD
Susanne E. Gionet, BS
Daniel J. Feller, PhD

SUMMARY. Benzodiazepine (BZ) effects include anxiolyis, sedation, seizure protection, and muscle relaxation; the mechanisms underlying these various effects are not understood. We have recently used the rotarod test in conjunction with selective breeding techniques to develop lines of mice which are diazepam-sensitive (DS) and diazepam-resistant (DR).* We review the general methods of selective breeding, along with a description of the DS/DR selection study, and then describe a variety of behavioral and neurochemical studies which have been conducted in an attempt to characterize these mice.

We have investigated the effects of other sedative drugs believed

---

Edward J. Gallaher is Research Pharmacologist, VA Medical Center, and Assistant Professor, Pharmacology and Medical Psychology at Oregon Health Sciences University, Portland, OR 97201. Susanne E. Gionet is Research Associate, VA Medical Center and Oregon Health Sciences University. Daniel J. Feller is Research Pharmacologist, VA Medical Center, and Assistant Professor, Pharmacology at Oregon Health Sciences University, Portland, OR 97201.

Send reprint requests to: Edward J. Gallaher, PhD, Research Service (151W), VA Medical Center, Portland, OR 97201.

This work was supported by the VA Medical Research Service and by USPHS Grant RO-1 NS23927.

The authors wish to thank Dr. Tamara J. Phillips for carefully reading the manuscript and making numerous helpful suggestions, and Dr. John K. Belknap for generously providing Figure 1.

---

*Limited numbers of DS and DR mice are available for collaborative studies. Contact Dr. Gallaher to determine availability and ongoing studies.

to interact with the BZ receptor, including ethanol, pentobarbital, and phenobarbital. We have also tested these mice for seizure threshold and open-field activity. DS and DR mice do not differ in diazepam-induced seizure protection, suggesting that different mechanisms underlie rotarod performance and the anti-convulsant effect. These results provide evidence to support the search for non-sedating anti-convulsants.

To determine the neurochemical basis for observed differences, BZ receptor density and chloride flux have been measured. We discuss the interaction between behavioral and neurochemical approaches, and describe a conceptual framework to guide future studies with these unique new animals.

INTRODUCTION

The benzodiazepines (BZs) are widely used clinically for their anxiolytic, sedative hypnotic, anti-convulsant, and muscle relaxant properties, and for some time were the most widely prescribed drugs world-wide.[1] In spite of their popularity, the mechanisms of action underlying these behavioral responses are poorly understood, and many questions remain that are relevant to clinical practice. For example, are each of these behavioral responses mediated by a single underlying mechanism? If multiple receptor types exist, might we be able to develop drugs which are more selective for one effect or another (e.g., non-sedating anxiolytics, or non-sedating anti-convulsants)? What are the mechanisms underlying the development of tolerance and physical dependence to the BZs? Does tolerance develop equally to each of these effects?

When introduced into clinical practice in 1960 the mechanism of action of the BZs was unknown. However, considerable progress has been made recently, and the field is developing rapidly. Briefly, several landmarks in BZ research include: (i) an awareness of gamma-aminobutyric acid (GABA) as the most important inhibitory transmitter in the CNS; GABA acts by increasing chloride influx to produce post-synaptic hyperpolarization;[2,3] (ii) electrophysiological studies which indicate that the BZs produce an increase in chloride influx via an intact GABA system;[4,5] (iii) the discovery of high-affinity stereospecific BZ receptors, including descriptions of their anatomical locations throughout the CNS;[6,7] and (iv) the recent cloning and sequencing of the GABA-BZ receptor/chloride ionophore complex.[8]

In the excitement generated by the sophisticated and powerful electrophysiological and molecular biology techniques described above, it must be kept in mind that the BZs are psychotropic drugs, administered for their effects on *behavior*. It is therefore essential that as molecular mechanisms are pursued, hypotheses and results are compared and correlated with the results of relevant animal models of behavior. In this paper we describe the selective breeding of unique lines of diazepam-sensitive (DS) and diazepam-resistant (DR) mice, which were developed to provide an animal model to facilitate such collaborative studies.[9]

Since selective breeding is becoming an increasingly important technique for producing animal models for behavioral and pharmacological research, we will briefly discuss underlying principles as we describe the development of DS and DR mice. We will then review some of the behavioral and neurochemical studies that have been conducted with DS and DR mice. Throughout this review we describe a conceptual framework which illustrates the potential role of selective breeding in the elucidation of drug mechanisms.

SELECTIVE BREEDING: THE DEVELOPMENT OF DS AND DR MICE

Our laboratory has long been interested in mechanisms of tolerance and physical dependence, and we were actively pursuing such studies with BZs.[10,11] During the course of this work we used a rotarod to monitor the discoordinating effects of sedative hypnotics. The rotarod is a horizontal, slowly rotating dowel, suspended above a bed of sawdust. Normally, a naive mouse can maintain its balance on the rotarod, but following the administration of ethanol, BZs, or other sedative hypnotics, the mouse falls off. This impairment persists until drug levels decline below some threshold concentration, at which time the animal regains its ability to perform the task. Upon injection with diazepam (10 mg/kg *per os*), we observed that some individuals were impaired longer than others. Although this might be due to differences in elimination rate, we further observed that those recovering early did so with higher brain BZ levels than those recovering later, suggesting a difference in CNS sensitivity to diazepam ($p < .001$; unpublished observations, Henauer and Gallaher).

The variation observed within a population may be partitioned into environmental and genetic factors. Environmental factors may include handling, location in the animal colony, order of testing, time of day, and maternal behavior, among many other possibilities. However, if at least some of the observed variation is due to genetic factors, then successive matings of sensitive individuals will lead to a segregation of genes, producing a new genotype which is on the average more sensitive than the original population. This technique has been widely used in agriculture and animal husbandry to develop commercial stocks which produce more eggs, more milk, sturdier offspring, and so on.[12] More recently these techniques have been extended to the behavioral research laboratory.[13]

We were aware of several prior selective breeding programs. For example, mice have been selected for ethanol-induced sleep time,[14] ethanol-induced physical dependence,[15] and opiate-induced analgesia.[16] However, no similar studies had been conducted with BZs. We postulated that it should be possible to selectively breed mice based on their sensitivity to diazepam, thereby producing sensitive and insensitive genetic stocks which would be available for a variety of behavioral and neurochemical studies.

A heterogeneous stock of mice (HS/Ibg) had been developed at the Institute for Behavioral Genetics in Boulder, CO by McClearn et al.[17] HS/Ibg mice were developed by a systematic cross-mating of individuals from eight inbred strains (A, BALB/c, C3H/2, C57BL, DBA/2, AKR, IS/Bi, and RIII) to produce animals having a broad mix of mouse genes. This foundation stock provides a rich genetic pool for the subsequent selection of genes which contribute to the trait in question.

In order to conduct a selective breeding program, a behavioral method is required to provide a graded measurement of drug sensitivity for each individual animal. A large number of animals are tested in a foundation population at selection generation S_0 (Figure 1). Males and females are then chosen from the sensitive extreme of the population and are mated to initiate the sensitive genotype. Likewise, individuals are chosen from the resistant extreme and mated to initiate the resistant genotype. The offspring (generation S_1) are tested; if there is a genetic component to the trait then we expect the mean of these two populations to differ. The extremes are again mated, producing generation S_2. If the trait is determined by a single genc, the sensitive and resistant lines will diverge maximally after a single generation. If the trait is polygenic the lines will diverge gradually. As all genes contributing to the trait are gradually segregated into the sensitive and resistant lines, the divergence between lines will reach a plateau.

Due to the large number of animals to be tested over the course of a selective breeding program it is advantageous to use a behavioral method which is quick and convenient, although this may not always be possible. Obviously, the test must also be non-lethal; for example, selection for seizure threshold would produce invaluable new genotypes, but the requirement for subsequent mating precludes such a selection criterion. (This is not strictly true, since techniques exist whereby siblings of the

FIGURE 1. Divergence of population means during a selective breeding program. Each curve illustrates a hypothetical frequency distribution describing the sensitivity of individuals within a population tested for a continuously varying trait. The abcissa indicates the value obtained for the trait; the ordinate indicates the relative frequency of animals performing at that level. In generation S_0, a single distribution is observed. The shaded areas indicate the individuals which are selected to serve as parents for the succeeding generation. In generation S_1, population means have diverged, but there is considerable overlap between the LO and HI lines. Again, extreme animals are chosen for mating. By generation S_3 there is little overlap between the HI and LO lines. (Figure courtesy JK Belknap.)

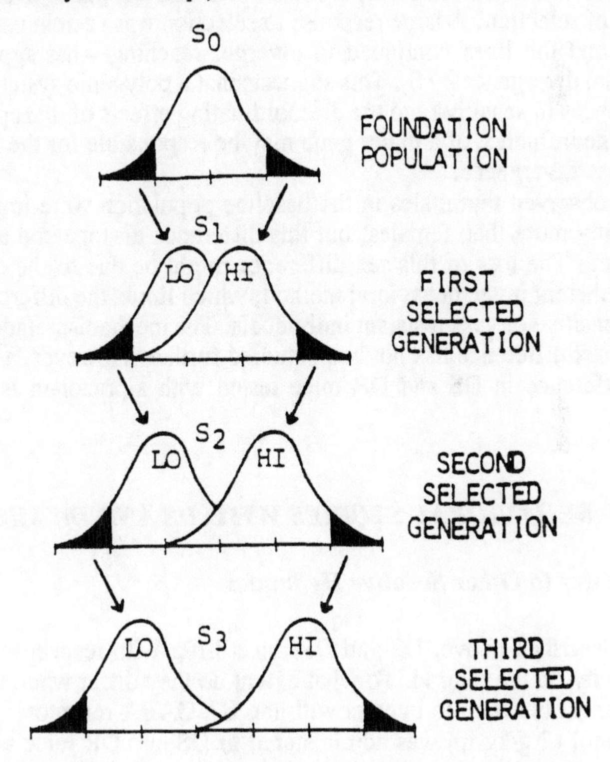

extreme animals may be mated. However, this technique is considerably less efficient since we do not have explicit information about the sensitivity of the individual animals which contribute to the next generation.)

We conducted pilot studies to determine an appropriate dose for loss of righting reflex, in an attempt to produce a BZ analog of long-sleep and short-sleep mice.[14] Surprisingly, doses ranging from 20 to 100 mg/kg did not produce a reliable loss of righting reflex. We therefore returned to the rotarod task. Although some investigators monitor the length of time that a mouse can remain on the fixed speed rotarod, we have found that more reliable results are obtained with a quantal test; that is, the mouse is scored pass/fail based on a 30-sec trial. Following the administration diazepam (20 mg/kg per os in corn oil), mice were tested every 10-15 min until they recovered the ability to perform (up to 300 min); the selection criterion was the duration of impairment from the time of injection. Figure 2 indicates the mean duration of impairment in DS and DR males over 13 generations of selection. A large response to selection was seen in early generations, and the lines continued to diverge, reaching what appears to be maximal divergence by S_5. This suggests that a polygenic system mediates differences in sensitivity to the discoordinating effects of diazepam. However, the influence of a major gene may be responsible for the large early response divergence.

We observed that males in the baseline population were impaired significantly more than females, but this difference disappeared as the lines diverged. The loss of this sex difference might be due to the ceiling and floor inherent in the behavioral method, which limits the differentiation of very sensitive or very resistant individuals. The mechanism underlying the initial sex difference has not been studied further. However, a remaining sex difference in DS and DR mice tested with alprazolam is described below.

BEHAVIORAL STUDIES WITH DS AND DR MICE

Sensitivity to Other Sedative Hypnotics

As described above, DS and DR mice differ with respect to diazepam sensitivity on the rotarod. To what extent do they differ when tested with other drugs believed to interact with the BZ-GABA receptor?

Ethanol (2 g/kg ip) was administered to DS and DR mice which were then tested on the rotarod until they regained their ability to perform the task; at this time tail blood samples were drawn to indicate blood ethanol concentrations (BECs). Male DR mice recovered in 41 min, with BECs of 1.85 mg/ml; DS mice recovered later (73 min), with lower BECs (1.49 mg/ml; $p < .01$). Most interesting, however, was the response of the two lines after five sequential ethanol injections. Over the course of the day, DR mice became quite tolerant, whereas DS mice became only slightly

FIGURE 2. Divergence in mean duration of rotarod impairment in DS and DR male mice over thirteen generations of selective breeding.

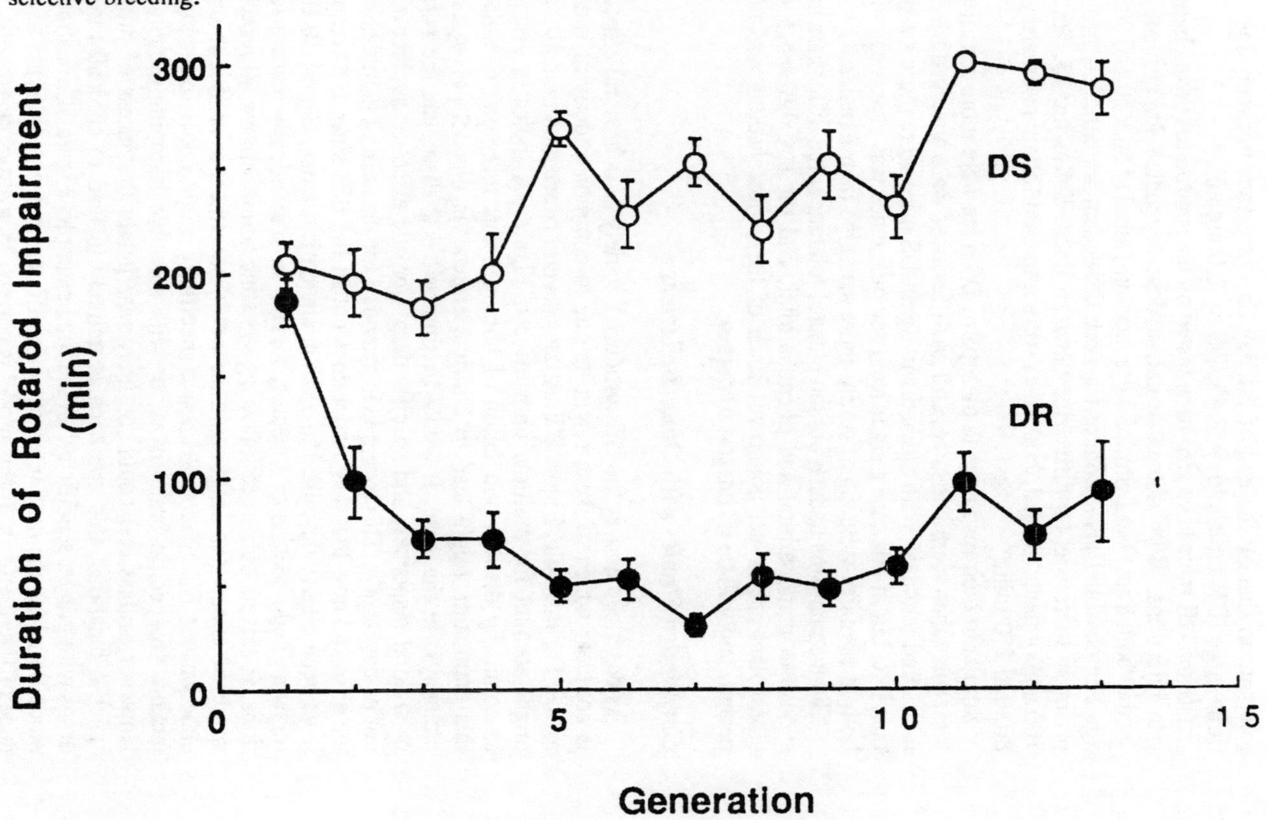

tolerant, so that by the end of the day the difference between lines was quite large (DR threshold = 3.45, DS = 2.0 mg/ml).[18]

DS and DR mice have also been tested on the rotarod following barbiturate injections. With phenobarbital, a dose-dependent impairment was seen in both lines, but DS mice were more impaired at both 50 and 70 mg/kg. Pentobarbital also produced a dose-dependent impairment, but surprisingly there was no difference between lines. Following 25, 50, and 100 mg/kg pentobarbital, both lines were impaired for approximately 40, 80, and 210 min.[19]

Similar to their responses to diazepam, DS mice were more sensitive to lorazepam than were DR mice, and no differences were observed between males and females. With alprazolam, again DS mice were more sensitive than DR, but in this case a significant sex difference was observed; within both lines males were significantly more sensitive than females.

The mechanisms underlying the ethanol tolerance, the difference in response to pentobarbital and phenobarbital, and the sex difference with alprazolam are as yet unknown. Each of these observations was unexpected, and will be of interest to pursue.

Correlative Studies with Other Behaviors

As described above, the BZs produce a variety of behavioral effects; it is not clear which of these might be due to common underlying mechanisms. For example, Figure 3 illustrates several conceptual models which might account for multiple drug effects. Figure 3A indicates a single, anatomically distinct population of homogeneous receptors; stimulating this population might lead to multiple effects via distinct post-synaptic pathways. In this case, it would be impossible to dissociate the various behavioral responses, and specific drugs for one effect or another could not be developed. This example is provided for the sake of completeness; we already know that this model does not fit the BZs since BZ receptors have been clearly described in distinct anatomical areas. Figure 3B illustrates a single species of receptor, located in anatomically distinct locations. In this model, since following systemic administration all receptors would be exposed to drug, again we would not expect to be able to dissociate various BZ effects. Response specificity might occur following injections to specific brain areas, or with selective lesioning techniques. However, unless one could routinely manipulate the access of drug to specific locations, this approach is unlikely to lead to clinically useful drugs with greater specificity. In the final example, Figure 3C illustrates a model in which the drug interacts with different receptor subtypes to produce different effects. If this model is correct, then structure-activity rela-

FIGURE 3. Schematic model of possible drug(D) - receptor(R) interactions leading to multiple observed behaviors. A. Drug acts on a homogeneous population of receptors in a single anatomical location, leading to multiple effects. This model precludes the development of receptor ligands which produce specific effects. B. Drug acts on homogeneous receptor populations, located in specific anatomical locations, leading to multiple effects. This model requires pharmacokinetic manipulation to elicit selective effects, since all receptors will be affected by systemic drug. C. Drug acts on heterogeneous receptor populations. This model provides promise for the development of drugs which are specific for one receptor subtype over another.

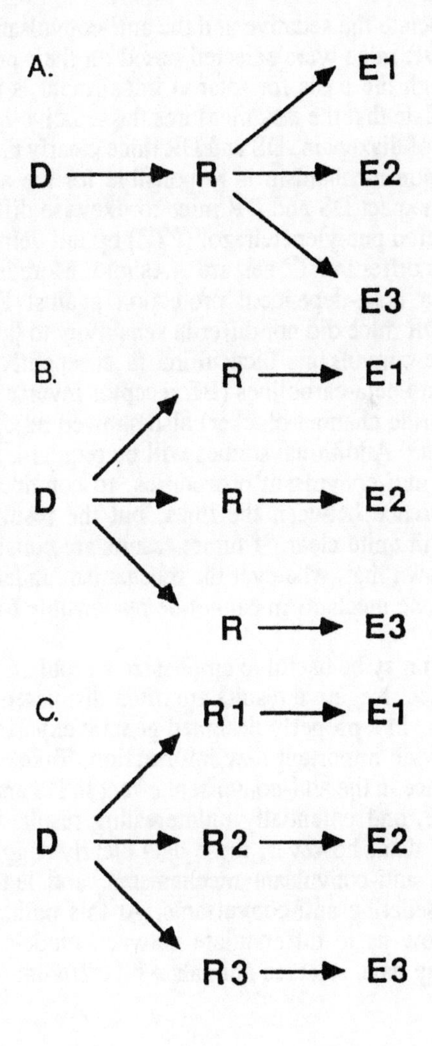

tionship studies would have a high probability of leading to drugs which would be specific to one or another receptor subtype. A considerable amount of neurochemical data, and a lesser amount of behavioral data exist to support such a model. The examples below illustrate the role that DS and DR mice may play in the process of differentiating the mechanisms underlying the various BZ effects.

Seizure Susceptibility and the Anti-convulsant Effect of Diazepam

Can we dissociate the sedative and the anti-convulsant effects of diazepam? DS and DR mice were selected based on their performance on the rotarod. Although the basis for rotarod impairment is not clearly understood, we postulate that the task measures the sedative-hypnotic or muscle relaxant effects of diazepam. DS and DR mice clearly differ on the rotarod task. If a common mechanism is responsible for the anti-convulsant effect, we would expect DS and DR mice to likewise differ on this test.

We administered pentylenetetrazol (PTZ) by tail vein infusion; DS and DR mice did not differ in PTZ seizure threshold. More importantly, diazepam produces a dose-dependent protection against PTZ seizures, but again, DS and DR mice did not differ in sensitivity to this effect.[20] Further studies with the convulsants bicuculline (a competitive GABA antagonist), DMCM and beta-carbolines (BZ receptor inverse agonists), and picrotoxin (a chloride channel blocker) also showed no difference between DS and DS lines.[21] Additional studies will be required, using a variety of convulsant and anti-convulsant procedures, to convince us that there is indeed no difference between the lines, but the results of these initial experiments seem quite clear. If future results are consistent, the conclusion must be drawn that, whatever the mechanism underlying rotarod impairment, the same mechanism cannot be responsible for the anti-convulsant effect.

At this point it may be useful to emphasize a problem in "selling" such correlative studies. Negative results are often dismissed as being uninteresting. However, in a properly designed genetic experiment, "negative" results may provide important new information. Taken alone, the failure to find a difference in the anti-convulsant effect in DS and DR lines appear to be a negative, and potentially uninteresting result. Considered along with the rotarod data, however, these data clearly suggest the separation of sedative and anti-convulsant mechanisms, and lend impetus to the search for non-sedating anti-convulsants. At this point, the data are not sufficient to allow us to differentiate between models 2B and 2C. For example, we may have selected animals with different numbers of receptors in critical anatomical locations. Conversely, we may have selected animals with qualitatively different receptor subtypes. These questions are pursued in the neurochemical experiments described below.

Open-Field Activity

Low doses of sedative hypnotics generally lead to arousal, perhaps observed as an increase in noise level at a cocktail party, or as an increase in motor activity in small animals monitored in an open-field apparatus. Phillips and Gallaher reported differences in open-field activity in DS and DR mice, with DR mice being *more* sensitive to the locomotor stimulant effects of diazepam.[22] In this test, activity was monitored by infrared photocells for 15 min. Following a vehicle injection, mean activity counts in both lines were approximately 650. Following 10 and 20 mg/kg diazepam, mean activity counts in DR mice increased to 1300-1500 counts. Activity decreased with higher doses (30-40 mg/kg), presumably as a result of sedation. In contrast, activity in DS mice *declined* slightly at all doses. A similar pattern was observed with flunitrazepam, except that a more profound inhibition of activity was seen in the DS line.

One interpretation of these data is that the low-dose activating effect of diazepam is masked by sedation in DS mice, whereas minimal sedation in DR mice allows the low-dose activating effect to be more readily observed. For example, it has been proposed that the low-dose activating effect of ethanol is mediated by dopaminergic systems, and that this effect is masked by the sedation resulting from higher doses.[23] The ambulatory effects of diazepam may be similarly mediated, albeit indirectly via GABA systems. DS and DR mice might serve as one animal model to test this hypothesis. If DS mice are more sensitive to BZ-GABA-induced sedation, then perhaps by antagonizing the sedative BZ effect with a competitive antagonist it will be possible to elicit activation in DS mice.

DS and DR mice were also tested in the open-field with ethanol, pentobarbital, and phenobarbital. With each of these drugs a dose-dependent activation was observed in both lines. Line differences were observed following ethanol and pentobarbital, with DR mice showing more activation. Following phenobarbital, dose-dependent activation was observed, but there was no line difference. Note that this disparity between pentobarbital and phenobarbital is opposite to the results obtained using the rotarod, suggesting that these drugs act via different mechanisms in producing these two effects.

Anxiolytic Effects of Benzodiazepines

The benzodiazepines are widely prescribed for their anxiolytic effect, and numerous animal models have been developed to screen anxiolytic drug effects. These tests can generally be placed into three classes: reward-conflict tests, exposure to a novel environment, and fear-enhanced startle. Preliminary studies are in progress in our laboratory to adapt several of these procedures from rats to mice, at which time DS and DR mice will be tested with a variety of anxiogenic and anxiolytic compounds. It will be of interest to determine which, if any, of these traits, have segregated into the divergent lines of mice. If DS and DR mice have not diverged with respect to anxiolytic effects, this will stimulate the search for the distinct mechanisms responsible for sedation and anxiolysis.

NEUROCHEMICAL STUDIES

As data continue to be collected with DS and DR mice, it will be of interest to compare behavioral results with data emanating from neurochemical and molecular biology laboratories.

Receptor Density and Affinity

Given the large difference in performance observed between DS and DR mice, we might expect that we have selected for mice with larger or smaller populations of BZ receptors, or conversely, that receptors are more or less sensitive to BZ-induced augmentation of GABA-induced chloride flux. Allan et al.[24] found no difference in the density or affinity of BZ receptors in whole brain assays conducted on DS and DR mice, using [^{3}H]-flunitrazepam and [^{35}S]-TBPS as ligands for the BZ site and the chloride channel, respectively. It is clear, however, that observation of small changes in specific receptor populations might well be masked by assaying whole brain. Therefore, we recently repeated the flunitrazepam binding study in specific brain areas as previously described by Feller et al.,[25] with some modifications. Binding was performed using a thoroughly washed crude membrane homogenate. Homogenate and increasing concentrations of [^{3}H]-flunitrazepam (0.08 - 8 nM) were incubated at 4° C for 150 min. The reaction was terminated by vacuum filtration over Whatman GF/B filters to separate bound from free drug. Non-specific binding was determined in the presence of 1 uM diazepam. The K_d and B_{max} values were determined using the computer program of McPherson[26] based on the method of Munson and Rodbard.[27] Table 1 indicates that no differences were observed in cortex, corpus striatum, hippocampus, cerebellum, or

TABLE 1

[^{3}H]-Flunitrazepam Binding in DS and DR Mice

	N	K_d (nM)		B_{max} (pmol/mg protein)	
		DS	DR	DS	DR
Cerebral Cortex	6	1.78±.05	1.70±.04	1.57±.15	1.38±.04
Corpus Striatum	6	1.29±.10	1.16±.04	1.97±.11	1.75±.14
Hippocampus	6	1.83±.13	1.71±.04	1.41±.06*	1.64±.06*
Cerebellum	6	1.90±.08	1.89±.04	0.66±.02	0.68±.02
Brain Stem	6	1.63±.08	1.31±.04	1.07±.10	1.07±.04

* $p < 0.05$

brain stem. Collectively, these results indicate that DS/DR sensitivity differences cannot easily be attributed to differences in BZ receptor binding characteristics, at least at this level of resolution.

Receptor Autoradiography

It is clear from the elegant quantitative autoradiographic work presented in this symposium by Belknap, that dissection of specific brain areas may still be inadequate for resolving small but potentially critical differences in receptor density. Belknap has shown that mice which are sensitive to opiate-induced analgesia have a small "hot-spot" of high receptor density in the dorsal portion of the dorsal raphe nucleus, whereas those that are resistant to this effect exhibit much reduced binding in this area.[28]

As a consequence of these studies we have initiated an autoradiographic survey of DS and DR mouse brains. In these studies we will determine the location and density of the various ligand binding sites associated with the BZ-GABA receptor complex. Further, as a consequence of the isolation and purification of various BZ receptor subunits, cDNA probes and monoclonal antibodies are being developed in various laboratories. In addition to determining ligand binding sites, these probes will make it possible to monitor the location and density of specific receptor subunits. It is possible that in selectively breeding mice for diazepam sensitivity, we have in fact selected for a preponderance of one receptor subtype over another. These new methods and probes provide an approach that should allow this question to be answered.

Chloride Flux

Another approach to determining the underlying difference between DS and DR mice is to monitor the *function* of the BZ-GABA receptor. This is accomplished by measuring $^{36}C1^{-}$ flux into isolated membrane microsacs containing the BZ-GABA receptor chloride ionophore.[29] Allan et al.[24] found muscimol, a GABA agonist, to be a more potent stimulator of $^{36}C1^{-}$ influx in DS compared to DR mice. In addition, flunitrazepam augmented muscimol-stimulated chloride influx in DS, but not in DR mice. However, no difference was observed in muscimol-stimulated flunitrazepam binding.

Studies with other sedative hypnotics indicated that ethanol augmented $^{36}C1^{-}$ influx in DS, but not DR mice, pentobarbital produced a similar dose-dependent increase in $1^{36}C1^{-}$ influx in both lines, and phenobarbital produced a dose-dependent influx, with DS microsacs being significantly more affected than DR microsacs. These results are remarkably consistent with the behavioral data described above. As in the case of the receptor binding studies, these experiments were conducted on microsacs from whole brains. Additional work will be required to determine if the observed differences are amplified in specific brain areas.

CONCLUSION

The benzodiazepines are clinically important drugs, and have been intensively studied over the past ten years, following reports of stereospecific high-affinity receptors. It is not clear which BZ effects are mediated by common underlying mechanisms, and this question is crucial for the development of specific drugs with minimal side effects. Following a number of exciting advances in psychopharmacology and molecular biology, we appear to be at the threshold of understanding the relationship between a specific CNS receptor system and the behavioral manifestations of manipulating this system.

We have described here the development of new lines of mice which are sensitive or resistant to benzodiazepines, and further describe a variety of behavioral and neurochemical studies conducted with these mice. Obviously, the work with these interesting animals has just begun.

REFERENCES

1. Parry HJ, Balter LB, Mellinger GD, Cissin IH, and Manheimer DI. National patterns of psychotherapeutic drug use. Arch Gen Psychiatry 1973; 28:769-783.

2. Martin IL. The benzodiazepines and their receptors: 25 years of progress. Neuropharmacology 1987; 26:957-970.

3. Haefely W, Kulcsar A, Mohler H, Pieri L, Polc P, and Schaffner R. Possible involvement of GABA in the central nervous actions of benzodiazepines. In: Mechanism of Action of Benzodiazepines, Costa E. and Greengard P., (eds.) New York, Raven Press, 1975, 131-151.

4. Schmidt RF, Vogel E, and Zimmermann M. Die wirkung von Diazepam auf die presynaptische Hemmung und andere Ruckenmarksreflexe. Naunyn-Schmied Arch Pharmacol. 1967; 258:69-82.

5. Polc P, Mohler H, and Haefely, W. The effect of diazepam on spinal cord activities: possible sites and mechanisms of actions. Naunyn-Schmied Arch Pharmacol. 1974; 284:319-337.

6. Mohler H and Okada T. Benzodiazepine receptor: demonstration in the central nervous system. Science 1977; 198:849-851.

7. Squires RF and Braestrup C. Benzodiazepine receptors in rat brain. Nature 1977; 266:732-734.

8. Schofield PR et al. Sequence and functional expression of the GABA receptor shows a ligand-gated receptor super-family. Nature 1987; 328:221-227.

9. Gallaher EJ, Hollister LE, Gionet SE, and Crabbe JC. Mouse lines selected for genetic differences in diazepam sensitivity. Psychopharmacology 1987; 93:25-30.

10. Gallaher EJ, Henauer SA, Jacques CJ, and Hollister LE. Benzodiazepine dependence in mice following ingestion of drug-containing food pellets. J Pharmacol Exp Ther. 1986; 237:462-467.

11. Henauer SA, Gallaher EJ, and Hollister LE. Long-lasting single-dose tolerance to neurologic deficits induced by diazepam. Psychopharmacology 1984; 82:161-163.

12. Falconer RS. *Introduction to Quantitative Genetics 2nd edition*, Ronald Longman Group Ltd., London. 1983.

13. Roberts, RC. Current perspectives on selective breeding: theoretical aspects. In: McClearn GE, Deitrich RA, and Erwin VG (eds.) *Development of Animal Models as Pharmacogenetic Tools*. USDHHS-NIAAA Research Monograph No. 6, US Government Printing Office, Washington D.C. 1981.

14. McClearn GE and Kakihana R. Selective breeding for ethanol sensitivity: Short-sleep and Long-sleep mice. In: McClearn GE, Deitrich RA, and Erwin VG (eds.) *Development of Animal Models as Pharmacogenetic Tools*. USDHHS-NIAAA Research Monograph No. 6, US Government Printing Office, Washington D.C. 1981.

15. Crabbe JC, Kosobud A, and Young E. Genetic selection for ethanol withdrawal severity: differences in replicate mouse lines. Life Sci. 1983; 33:955-962.

16. Belknap JK, Haltli N, Goebel D, Lame M. Selective breeding for high and low levels of opiate-induced analgesia in mice. Behav Genetics 1983; 13:383-396.

17. McClearn GE, Wilson JY, and Meredith W. The use of isogenic and heterogenic mouse stocks in behavioral research. In: *Contributions to behavior–genetic analysis–the mouse as a prototype*. New York: Appleton-Century-Crofts, 1970:3-22.

18. Gallaher EJ and Gionet SE. Initial sensitivity and tolerance to ethanol in mice genetically selected for diazepam sensitivity. Alcoholism: Clin Exp Res. 1988; 12:77-80.

19. Gallaher EJ, Gionet SE, and Hollister LE. The effect of various sedative hypnotics on mice selectively bred for diazepam sensitivity. Pharmacologist 1986; 28:129.

20. Gallaher EJ and Gionet SE. Seizure thresholds in diazepam-sensitive and -resistant mice. Society Neurosci. Abstr. 1988; 14:350.

21. Gallaher EJ and Gionet SE. Effect of GABA-benzodiazepine receptor ligands on seizure threshold in diazepam-sensitive and -resistant mice. Society Neuroscience Abstr. 1989; 15:668.

22. Phillips TJ and Gallaher EJ. Ethanol and diazepam effects on locomotor activity in mice selectively bred for diazepam sensitivity. In Kuriyama D, Takada A, and Ishii H (eds.) *Biomedical and Social Aspects of Alcohol and Alcoholism*. New York, Excerpta Medica, 1988: 251-254.

23. Engel J and Liljequist S. The involvement of different central neurotransmitters in mediating the stimulatory and sedative effects of ethanol. In: Pohorecky L and Brick J (eds.) *Stress and Alcohol Use*. New York: Elsevier, 1983: 154-169.

24. Allan AM, Gallaher EJ, Gionet SE, and Harris RA. Genetic selection for benzodiazepine ataxia produces functional changes in the gamma-aminobutyric acid receptor chloride channel complex. Brain Res. 1988; 452:118-126.

25. Feller DJ, Harris RA, and Crabbe JC. Differences in GABA activity between ethanol withdrawal seizure prone and resistant mice. Eur J Pharmacol. 1988; 157: 147-154.

26. McPherson GA. Analysis of radioligand binding experiments: A collection of programs for the IBM PC. J Pharmacol Meth. 1985; 14:213-218.

27. Munson PJ and Rodbard D. A versatile computerized approach for the characterization of ligand binding systems. Anal. Biochem. 1980; 107:220-239.

28. *Belknap JK NIDA Technical Review 1989 (THESE PROCEEDINGS)*.

29. Harris AR and Allan AM. Functional coupling of GABA receptors to chloride channels in brain membranes. Science 1985; 228: 1108-1110.

Animal Models for the Study of Alcoholism: Utility of Selected Lines

J. C. Froehlich, PhD
T.-K. Li, MD

SUMMARY. One recent advance in the field of alcohol research has been the recognition that a predisposition to develop alcoholism is, in part, genetically determined. It now remains to identify the factors, which, when inherited, increase risk for alcoholism. One approach to this problem is to analyze how organisms with identifiable genetic predisposition towards ethanol drinking differ from organisms without genetic risk. Such an approach may lead to the identification of neurochemical, neurophysiological or neuroanatomical factors which, when inherited alone, or in combination, serve to predispose an organism towards ethanol drinking.

Genetic selection for ethanol preference or nonpreference has resulted in the derivation of rat lines which differ widely in oral ethanol intake. These rat lines represent animal models with multifaceted utility. Genetically selected lines are currently being used to: (1) identify heritable physiological characteristics which are associated with, and may be causally related to, differences in ethanol intake, (2) test for true genetic association between ethanol drinking and other ethanol-related traits and, (3)

J. C. Froehlich is affiliated with the Department of Medicine and the Department of Physiology/Biophysics, Indiana University School of Medicine, Indianapolis. T.-K. Li is affiliated with the Department of Medicine and the Department of Biochemistry, Indiana University School of Medicine, Indianapolis, IN 46202.

Address reprint requests to: J. C. Froehlich, Department of Medicine, 421 Emerson Hall, Indiana University School of Medicine, 545 Barnhill Drive, Indianapolis, IN 46202.

The research was supported, in part, by grants AA03243, AA07611 and AA07867 from the PHS.

investigate the efficacy of pharmacological, environmental and behavioral manipulations which have the potential to inhibit ethanol drinking. Examples of potentially promising associations of ethanol drinking behavior are sensitivity to the rewarding properties of ethanol, and tolerance to the aversive effects of ethanol. Several directions for further research are suggested.

One of the most interesting new developments in the field of alcohol research has been the recognition that excessive alcohol drinking, as well as many physiological and behavioral responses to alcohol are, at least in part, genetically determined. The demonstration that genetic factors contribute to the development of alcoholism has raised a fundamental question: "What exactly is inherited?" Identification of the biological and environmental variables that promote and maintain excessive alcohol drinking is key to our understanding of the disorder we call alcoholism. Currently very little is known about the specific processes and pathways that promote alcohol drinking in humans. When trying to identify the pharmacological, biochemical and neuroendocrine factors that may contribute to excessive alcohol drinking it is useful to have an animal model of alcoholism that permits the use of invasive experimental approaches which cannot be used in humans for ethical reasons.[1,10]

The problem with developing an animal model of alcoholism is that most lower animals, unlike man, do not usually drink enough alcohol to produce significant concentrations of alcohol in the blood.[1] However, there is a large degree of variability in the amount of alcohol that individual animals will consume. Although most rats within a given population drink very little alcohol when given a free-choice between alcohol and water, some rats will drink large amounts of alcohol. This individual variation in oral alcohol preference was first noted by Richter and Campbell,[2] and was subsequentially demonstrated in inbred mouse strains by McClearn and Rogers.[3]

When it was recognized that a propensity towards alcohol-drinking was, in part, heritable, it became clear that genetic pressure could be used to shift alcohol-drinking in animal populations. Eriksson, in Finland,[4] Mardones, in Chile[5] and Li and Lumeng in the U.S.[6] have subsequently demonstrated that rodents which differ widely in alcohol intake can be bidirectionally selected and bred to produce lines with very high or very low levels of voluntary alcohol consumption. Application of this genetic selection approach has resulted in the derivation of three pairs of rat lines which demonstrate either high or low alcohol preference: (1) the AA (Alko-Alcohol) and ANA (Alko-Nonalcohol) rat lines[7] (2) the UChA (low alcohol preference) and UChB (high alcohol preference) rat lines[8] and (3) the P (alcohol-preferring) and NP (alcohol-nonpreferring) rat lines.[9]

Rat lines which have been selected for high and low alcohol drinking are extremely useful for a number of reasons. First, they provide unique models for the exploration of biological and environmental variables that promote and maintain high or low alcohol drinking behavior. Second, they can be used to test for the presence of a true genetic correlation between alcohol drinking and other alcohol-related traits such as alcohol sensitivity, alcohol tolerance and the efficacy of alcohol as a reinforcer. Once a cluster of traits have been identified which correlate with high alcohol drinking, the possibility of a causal relationship between these traits and alcohol drinking can be examined. Third, rat lines which have been selected for high alcohol drinking, such as the P line, can be used to investigate the efficacy of pharmacological, environmental and behavioral manipulations which may have the therapeutic potential to inhibit excessive alcohol intake.

The application of selective breeding techniques to study biochemical and behavioral responses to alcohol is well established and represents one of the major advances in the field of alcohol research. Experience with this technique has resulted in an increased awareness of the need for proper genetic control and the utility of replicate lines.[10] When trying to identify traits that are associated with the trait selected for, it is crucial to have replicate lines that are selected for the same trait as was the original line. The appearance of an associated trait in both the original and the replicate lines powerfully decreases the likelihood that the observed relationship is fortuitous. As we shall see, in the case of the P and NP lines which were selected for high and low voluntary ethanol intake, line differences in a variety of ethanol-related traits such as ethanol sensitivity and ethanol tolerance have appeared in both the original and replicate lines.

DERIVATION OF THE P, NP, HAD AND LAD RAT LINES

In 1974, Li and Lumeng began a selective breeding program for high and low oral ethanol preference which has resulted in the derivation of the alcohol-preferring (P) and alcohol-nonpreferring (NP) rat lines.[6,11,12] The P and NP lines were developed through mass selection from a foundation stock of "outbred" Wistar rats from the Walter Reed Army Institute of Research. Rats were tested for ethanol preference during 4 days of access to ethanol alone followed by 4 weeks of free-choice between a 10% (v/v) ethanol solution and water with food available *ad libitum*. Rats were selected for breeding based on their average ethanol intake during the 4 weeks of free-choice between ethanol and water. Animals selected for breeding in the alcohol-preferring or P line were those that consumed ethanol in excess of 5 g ethanol/kg body weight/day and demonstrated a greater than 2:1 preference ratio for ethanol over water. Rats selected for breeding in the alcohol-nonpreferring or NP line were those that consumed less than 1.5 g/kg/day and did not exceed an ethanol to water preference ratio of 0.2:1. By the third generation of genetic selection, separation between the P and NP lines in terms of ethanol intake began to emerge. The P and NP lines are currently in the 31st and 30th generations of selection for ethanol preference or nonpreference respectively. Voluntary ethanol consumption (g/kg/day) during ethanol preference testing averages approximately 9.2 (± S.E. of 0.4) in the P line and 1.9 (± S.E. of 0.7) in the NP line. When presented with a free-choice between water and a 10% (v/v) ethanol solution with food freely available, rats of the P line consume approximately 20-30% of their total daily calories as ethanol by substituting ethanol calories for food calories. They maintain body weight at levels comparable to P rats given free access to food and water alone.[6,12]

Recognition of the importance of replicate lines led to the initiation of another selective breeding experiment for high and low alcohol preference by the Indiana group which has resulted in the derivation of four new replicate rat lines. These lines are designated as the high alcohol drinking (HAD-1 and HAD-2) and low alcohol drinking (LAD-1 and LAD-2) lines.[13] Because the P and NP lines originated from a limited genetic base, the HAD and LAD lines were selected from a foundation stock of the genetically heterogeneous N/Nih rat[14] which was developed from the systematic crossing of 8 separate inbred strains. Rats of the HAD and LAD lines were bred using within-family selection with eight families per line and a rotational breeding design to avoid subline formation. All rats were tested for oral ethanol preference and were selected for breeding using criteria similar to those used in the derivation of the P and NP rat lines. By the 3rd to 4th generation of selection, there was a clear divergence in voluntary ethanol intake between the HAD and LAD lines.[13] Rats of the HAD and LAD lines are currently in the 11th generation of selection for high or low oral ethanol intake. Voluntary ethanol consumption (g/kg/day) during ethanol preference testing averages approximately 7.1 (± S.E. of 0.5) in the HAD line and 1.4 (± S.E. of 0.3) in the LAD line.

Animals that exhibit abnormally intense alcohol-seeking behavior (vide infra), such as rats of the P and HAD lines, represent unique models that can be used to explore the biological and environmental factors which contribute to excessive alcohol drinking and to identify alcohol-related traits. Rats of the P line have been well-characterized over the past 15 years and comparison of the P and NP lines has resulted in the identification of a number of traits that are associated with high oral consumption of alcohol. The neurochemical traits which are associated with high alcohol drinking in rats of the P line have been discussed in detail elsewhere.[13-22] We will focus on the behavioral traits associated with oral alcohol preference.

BEHAVIORAL CHARACTERIZATION OF THE P AND NP LINES

Oral Alcohol Consumption

Rats of the P line voluntarily drink ethanol solutions ranging from 10-30% in sufficient quantities to produce pharmacologically meaningful blood alcohol concentrations (BACs) of 40-210 mg% when food and water are available *ad libitum*.[11,13,23] Chronic voluntary ethanol consumption by rats of the P line results in the development of ethanol tolerance and physical dependence.[13,24,25] Of major interest was the finding that when rats of the P and NP lines were compared, P rats develop within-session tolerance more quickly and remain tolerant longer than rats of the NP line.[26,27]

Reinforcing Properties of Alcohol

The classical definitions of a positive reinforcer include "any stimulus that strengthens the behavior upon which it is made contingent"[28] or "a stimulus event which, if it occurs in the proper temporal relation with a response, tends to maintain or to increase the strength of a response. . . ."[29] Thus, self-administration of a substance defines that substance as a reinforcer. It follows that any substance that is repeatedly self-administered can be said to have a strong reinforcing efficacy.

The P and NP lines were selected for breeding based on their demonstrated preference or nonpreference, respectively, for oral consumption of a 10% (v/v) ethanol solution, a concentration that is aversive to most rats. A genetic difference in oral ethanol preference may reflect a difference in the reinforcing properties of ethanol. This possibility has been investigated in a number of behavioral comparisions of the P and NP lines. Rats of the P line will work, through operant responding, to obtain ethanol in concentrations as high as 30%.[30,31] In a more detailed study, the behavior of rats from the P and NP lines was compared in an operant chamber where food was freely available but the animals were required to obtain all of their daily fluid through bar-pressing for either water or an ethanol solution. The concentration of the available ethanol solution ranged from 2-30% (v/v).[32] It was found that rats of the P line bar-press for ethanol over water at all of the ethanol concentrations tested. In contrast, rats of the NP line bar-press more for ethanol than for water only at low ethanol concentrations of 2% and 5%. At ethanol concentrations of 10% or higher, rats of the NP line bar-press predominately for water. These results suggest that rats of the P and NP lines differ in sensitivity to ethanol's reinforcing properties.

It is generally accepted that the action of ethanol is biphasic: reinforcing or rewarding at low blood ethanol concentrations, and aversive at moderate to high blood ethanol concentrations.[33] The reinforcing efficacy of low dose ethanol and the aversive strength of high dose ethanol has recently been explored in rats of the P and NP lines using a conditioned taste aversion (CTA) paradigm.[34] Four doses of ethanol, administered ip, were paired with the consumption of a 0.1% saccharin solution in rats from the P and NP lines. Repeated pairings of saccharin and ethanol in a dose of 1.0 g/kg produced stronger and more prolonged aversion to saccharin in NP rats, compared with P rats, at comparable blood ethanol levels. A low dose of ethanol (0.25 g/kg) produced transient conditioned facilitation of saccharin consumption in P rats, but not in NP rats, at comparable blood ethanol levels. These results indicate that rats of the P line find moderate doses of ethanol to be less aversive than do rats of the NP line and suggest that low doses of ethanol may be reinforcing for rats of the P but not the NP line.

In the CTA paradigm, ethanol was administered ip thereby bipassing the oral cues, such as taste and smell, which accompany alcohol drinking. The results suggest that the rewarding and aversive properties of ethanol result from ethanol's postingestional effects rather than from orosensory cues. This conclusion agrees well with a previous finding that rats of the P line, but not the NP line, self-administer significant quantities of ethanol intragastrically.[30,31]

The results of the CTA study suggest that the postabsorptive effects of low dose ethanol are more reinforcing for rats of the P line than for those of the NP line. This interpretation is strengthened by the finding that low dose ethanol produces more behavioral stimulation in P rats than in NP rats as measured by spontaneous motor activity.[35] It is possible, therefore, that ingestion of small amounts of ethanol by rats of the P line produces reinforcing pharmacological effects which increase the probability of subsequent drinking. The results of the behavioral experiments performed to date indicate that rats of the P line have enhanced responsiveness to the low-dose reinforcing effects of ethanol, less aversion to moderate doses of ethanol, are able to develop tolerance to the aversive effects of ethanol more rapidly and to maintain tolerance longer than rats of the NP line. The increased potency of low-dose ethanol as a reinforcer for rats of the P line might be expected to foster and maintain ethanol drinking. Weaker aversion to the pharmacological effects of high doses of ethanol in the P line would allow P rats to drink more ethanol than NP rats before the postingestional effects become aversive. Rapid induction of tolerance to the aversive effects of ethanol with repeated bouts of voluntary ethanol drinking, as well as persistence of ethanol tolerance in rats of the P line might then serve to increase and maintain alcohol seeking behavior. We suggest that these are powerful mechanisms that may serve to promote and maintain ethanol self-administration.

GENERALITY OF ETHANOL-RELATED TRAITS

Recent studies have indicated that rats of the HAD line are similar to those of the P line in terms of many ethanol-related traits. For instance, rats of the HAD line will work on operant schedules for ethanol reward with ethanol concentrations as high as 30%. As was found in the NP rats, LAD rats have a very low response rate on operant schedules for ethanol reward when ethanol concentrations exceed 5%.[36] In addition, in parallel with the findings in the P and NP lines, HAD rats remain tolerant to the sedative/hypnotic effects of high dose ethanol longer than do rats of the LAD line.[37] We continue to find that many of the traits that were associated with ethanol preference and high ethanol intake in the P line are associated with ethanol preference in the HAD line as well. Such replication moves us significantly closer to establishing a true association between ethanol drinking and other traits such as ethanol sensitivity and ethanol tolerance. The extent to which each of these associated traits contributes to excessive ethanol drinking remains to be determined. Establishing trait causality will entail identification of the trait or traits that are necessary and sufficient for the emergence of abnormal alcohol seeking behavior. Given that both environmental factors and genetically determined biological traits contribute to excessive ethanol intake, the task of identifying the combination of genetic traits and environmental events which together will invariably produce excessive alcohol drinking is formidable. This is our challenge.

FUTURE DIRECTIONS

The most obvious use for genetic models is the identification of heritable traits. This emphasis on heritability can result in a focus on identifying biological rather than environmental factors which contribute to alcohol drinking. Given that the P, NP, HAD and LAD lines were derived by genetic selection, it is not surprising that much of the research on these rat lines has involved identifying neurochemical and neuroendocrine factors which may result in a predisposition towards excessive ethanol drinking. However, these genetically selected rat lines can also be used to explore environmental factors which can facilitate or inhibit ethanol drinking behavior.[38] We are interested in identifying environmental manipulations which can be used to decrease ethanol intake in the face of a genetic load that predisposes the animal towards ethanol drinking. Recently we have also begun to identify environmental events and conditions that have the potential of increasing chronic ethanol intake in rats that have no identifiable genetic predisposition towards ethanol drinking.[39,40] These types of investigations should provide valuable insights into the motivation for drinking which could then be used in the classification and treatment of individuals who use and abuse alcohol.

REFERENCES

1. Cicero TJ. A critique of animal analogues of alcoholism. In: Majchrowicz E and Noble EP ed. Biochemistry and Pharmacology of Ethanol, Vol 2. New York: Plenum Publishing Co, 1979; 533-560.
2. Richter CP and Campbell KH. Alcohol taste thresholds and concentrations of solution preferred by rats. Science, 1940; 91:507-508.
3. McClearn GE and Rodgers DA. Differences in alcohol preference among inbred strains of mice. J Stud Alcohol. 1959; 20:691-695.
4. Eriksson K. Genetic selection for voluntary alcohol consumption in the albino rat. Science 1968; 159:739-741.
5. Mardones J. Experimentally induced changes in the free selection of ethanol. Internat Rev Neurobiol. 1960; 2:41-76.
6. Lumeng L, Hawkins TD and Li T-K. New strains of rats with alcohol preference and nonpreference. In: Thurman, RG, Williamson, JR, Drott, HR and Chance B, eds. Alcohol and Aldehyde Metabolizing Systems. New York: Academic Press, 1977; 3:537-544.
7. Eriksson K and Rusi M. Finnish selection studies on alcohol-related behaviors: General outline. In: McClearn GE, Deitrich RA and Erwin VG, eds. NIAAA Research Monograph-6. Development of Animal Models as Pharmacogenetic Tools. Washington D.C.: U.S. Government Printing Office, 1981.

8. Mardones J and Segozia-Riquelene N. Thirty-two years of selection of rats by ethanol preference: UChA and UChB strains. Neurobehav Toxicol Teratol. 1983; 5:171-178.

9. Lumeng L, Li T-K, McBride WJ, Murphy JM, Morzorati SL and Froehlich JC. Mechanism(s) of modulation of alcohol consumption: Studies on the P and NP rats. Clifton, New Jersey: Humana Press, 1989; 359-370.

10. Crabbe JC. Genetic animal models in the study of alcoholism. Alcoholism: Clin Exper Res. 1989; 13:120-127.

11. Li T-K, Lumeng L, McBride WJ and Waller MB. Progress toward a voluntary oral consumption model of alcoholism. Drug and Alcohol Dep. 1979; 4:45-60.

12. Li T-K, Lumeng L, McBride WJ and Waller MB. Indiana selection studies on alcohol-related behaviors. In: McClearn GE, Deitrich RA and Erwin VG, eds. Development of Animal Models as Pharmacogenetic Tools. National Institute on Alcohol Abuse and Alcoholism Research Monograph 1981; 6:171-191.

13. Lumeng L, Doolittle DP and Li T-K. New duplicate lines of rats that differ in voluntary alcohol consumption. Alcohol and Alcoholism, 1986; 21:A125.

14. Hansen C and Spuhler K. Development of the National Institutes of Health genetically heterogeneous rat stock. Alcoholism: Clin Exp Res. 1984; 8:477-479.

15. Murphy JM, McBride WJ, Lumeng L and Li T-K. Regional brain levels of monoamines in alcohol-preferring and -nonpreferring lines of rats. Pharmacol Biochem Behav. 1982; 16:145-149.

16. Murphy JM, McBride WJ, Lumeng L and Li T-K. Contents of monoamines in forebrain regions of alcohol-preferring (P) and nonpreferring (NP) lines of rats. Pharmacol Biochem Behav. 1987; 26:389-392.

17. Froehlich JC, Harts J, Lumeng L and Li T-K. Naloxone attenuation of voluntary alcohol consumption. Alcohol and Alcoholism. 1987; 1:333-337.

18. Froehlich JC, Harts J, Lumeng L and Li T-K. Enkephalinergic involvement in voluntary ethanol consumption. Excerpta Medica International Congress Series 1988; 805:235-238.

19. Li T-K, Lumeng L, Doolittle DP, McBride WJ, Murphy JM, Froehlich JC and Morzorati S. Behavioral and neurochemical associations of alcohol-seeking behavior. Excerpta Medica International Congress Series, 1988; 805:435-438.

20. Li T-K, Lumeng L, McBride WJ, Murphy JM, Froehlich JC and Morzorati S. Pharmacology of alcohol preference in rodents. In: Stimmel B, ed. Advances in Alcohol and Substance Abuse. New York: Haworth Press, 1988:73-86.

21. Froehlich JC and Li T-K. Enkephalinergic involvement in voluntary alcohol drinking. In: Reid L., ed. Opioids, Bulimia, Alcohol Abuse and Alcoholism. Springer-Verlag Publishing Company, 1989; 217-228.

22. Froehlich JC, Harts J, Lumeng L and Li T-K. Naloxone attenuates ethanol intake in rats selectively bred for high ethanol preference. Pharm Biochem Beh. 1990; 35:385-390.

23. Murphy JM, Gatto GJ, Waller MB, McBride WJ, Lumeng L and Li T-K. Effects of scheduled access on ethanol intake by the alcohol-preferring P line of rats. Alcohol, 1986; 3:331-336.

24. Gatto GJ, Murphy JM, Waller MB, McBride WJ, Lumeng L and Li T-K. Chronic ethanol tolerance through free-choice drinking in the P line of alcohol-preferring rats. Pharmacol Biochem Behav. 1987; 28:111-115.

25. Waller MB, McBride WJ, Lumeng L and Li T-K. Induction of dependence on ethanol by free-choice drinking in alcohol-preferring rats. Pharmacol Biochem Behav. 1982; 16:501-507.

26. Waller MB, McBride WJ, Lumeng L and Li T-K. Initial sensitivity and acute tolerance to ethanol in the P and NP lines of rats. Pharmacol Biochem Behav. 1983; 19:683-686.

27. Gatto GJ, Murphy JM, Waller MB, McBride WJ, Lumeng L and Li T-K. Persistence of tolerance to a single dose of ethanol in the selectively bred alcohol-preferring P rats. Pharmacol Biochem Behav. 1987; 28:105-110.

28. Skinner BF. Punishment. In: BF Skinner, Science and Human Behavior. New York: Collier Macmillan Publishers, 1953:184-186.

29. Hulse SH, Egeth H and Deese J. The Psychology of Learning. New York: McGraw-Hill, 1980.

30. Penn PE, McBride WJ, Lumeng L, Gaff TM and Li T-K. Neurochemical and operant behavioral studies of a strain of alcohol-preferring rats. Pharmacol Biochem Behav. 1978; 8:475-481.

31. Waller MB, McBride WJ, Gatto GJ, Lumeng L and Li T-K. Intragastric self-infusion of ethanol by the P and NP (alcohol-preferring and -nonpreferring) lines of rats. Science, 1984; 225:78-80.

32. Murphy JM, Gatto GJ, McBride WJ, Lumeng L and Li T-K. Operant responding for oral ethanol in the alcohol-preferring P and alcohol-nonpreferring NP lines of rats. Alcohol, 1989; 6:127-131.

33. Pohorecky LA. Biphasic action of ethanol. Biobehav Rev. 1977; 1:231-240.

34. Froehlich JC, Harts J, Lumeng L and Li T-K. Differences in response to the aversive properties of ethanol in rats selectively bred for oral ethanol preference. Pharm Biochem Behav 1988; 32:215-222.

35. Waller MB, Murphy JM, McBride WJ, Lumeng L and Li T-K. Effect of low dose ethanol on spontaneous motor activity in alcohol-preferring and -nonpreferring lines of rats. Pharmacol Biochem Behav. 1986; 24:617-625.

36. Levy AD, McBride WJ, Murphy J, Lumeng L and Li T-K. Genetically selected lines of high- and low-alcohol-drinking rats: operant studies. Abs Soc Neurosci. 1988; 14:41.

37. Froehlich JC, Hostetler J, Lumeng L and Li T-K. Association between alcohol preference and acute tolerance. Alcohol, 1989; under editorial review.

38. Li T-K, Lumeng L, Froehlich JC, Murphy JM and McBride WJ. Genetic influence on response to the reinforcing properties of ethanol in rats. Excerpta Medica International Congress Series, 1988; 805:477-480.

39. Samson HH, Tolliver GA, Lumeng L and Li T-K. Ethanol reinforcement in the alcohol-nonpreferring (NP) rat: Initiation using behavioral techniques without food restriction. Alcoholism: Clin Exp Res. 1989; 13:378-385.

40. Gatto GJ, Murphy JM, McBride WJ, Lumeng L and Li T-K. Effects of fluoxetine and desipramine on palatability-induced ethanol consumption in the alcohol-nonpreferring (NP) line of rats. Alcohol, 1989; under editorial review.

Use of Recombinant Inbred Strains to Assess Vulnerability to Drug Abuse at the Genetic Level

Tamara J. Phillips, PhD
John K. Belknap, PhD
John C. Crabbe, PhD

SUMMARY. The use of Recombinant Inbred mouse Strains (RIS) to derive information about the complexity of the genetic architecture underlying various traits is increasing in popularity. Behaviors measured to index sensitivity to drug effects and vulnerability to drug abuse are considered here. Potential uses of RIS are identification of major gene effects, mapping of traits to particular chromosomal sites, determining genetic correlations between characters, and identifying behaviorally extreme genotypes. This approach has led to identification of a major gene moderating alcohol acceptance in mice and has revealed a more complex polygenic system influencing morphine consumption.

Tamara J. Phillips and John C. Crabbe are affiliated with the Research Service, VA Medical Center, and the Departments of Medical Psychology and Pharmacology, Oregon Health Sciences University, Portland, OR 97201. John K. Belknap is affiliated with the Departments of Pharmacology and Neuroscience, University of North Dakota, School of Medicine, Grand Forks, ND and the Research Service, VA Medical Center, and the Departments of Medical Psychology and Pharmacology, Oregon Health Sciences University, Portland, OR 97201.

Reprint requests should be mailed to: Tamara J. Phillips, PhD, Research Geneticist, Veterans Administration Medical Center, Research Service (151-W), 3710 S.W. U.S. Veterans Hospital Rd., Portland, OR 97201.

The authors wish to acknowledge Kim Sampson and Gayle Aasen who provided very able technical assistance for the morphine consumption studies.

This work was supported by PHS grant DA 02723, NIDA Contract 271-87-8120, and two grants from the Department of Veterans Affairs.

A powerful genetic animal model for detecting single gene effects and genetic correlations is advancing in familiarity and utilization in the study of abused drugs. D.W. Bailey[1] developed a set of Recombinant Inbred mouse Strains (RIS) for use in immunological research, but it has since been recognized that this methodology can be adapted to a variety of research fields concerned with genetic mediation. The study of genetically-determined sensitivity to drugs and of genetic vulnerability to drug abuse are not exceptions.

DEVELOPMENT OF RECOMBINANT INBRED STRAINS (RIS)

RIS development requires a sequence of breeding events. First, two highly inbred progenitor strains are interbred to produce a genetically identical F_1 population in which each individual carries a copy of each progenitor-type allele at every gene locus. Next, the F_1s are randomly bred to produce the genetically heterogeneous F_2 generation. Finally, randomly chosen brother-sister pairs from the F_2 generation are inbred to homozygosity at each locus (20 generations or more) resulting in some number of RIS determined by the original number of chosen pairs and by survival (reproductive success). Any loci polymorphic in the two progenitor strains will undergo segregation and independent assortment in their F_2 generation, and inbreeding of F_2 pairs will lead to fixation in the homozygous state of a particular allele at each locus in each RIS. Barring mutation, the fixed allele at each locus must come from one of the progenitor strains. Each RIS, therefore, represents the genetic fixation of a random sample of the genetic variance available by recombination in the F_2 generation, and potentially important gene combinations, different from those present in the parental strains, may occur in the RIS.

THEORY AND UTILIZATION OF RIS IN PHARMACOGENETIC RESEARCH

As alluded to above, RIS provide an especially powerful tool for establishing genetic associations, identifying major gene effects, and for chromosomal gene mapping once a major gene effect has been detected. An RIS analysis of a phenotype is most likely to be interesting and informative when the two progenitor strains differ markedly for that phenotype. In this case, the RIS battery derived from those strains may be tested and a Strain Distribution Pattern (SDP) established. The most exciting outcome is a bimodal distribution of the RIS responses, when each RIS resembles one of the progenitor strains, because such an outcome suggests the important influence of a single gene. An example of such an outcome is presented by Jeste et al.[2] in a pharmacogenetic analysis of the effect of B-phenylethylamine (PEA), an amphetamine-like drug, on locomotor activity. They tested the two progenitor strains, C57BL/6By (B6/By) and BALB/cBy (C/By), their two reciprocal F_1 hybrids, and the 7 RIS derived from these progenitors. PEA reduced the activity of B6/By mice and had no effect on the activity of C/By mice compared to the activity of saline control groups. Both F_1 hybrids responded like B6/By mice as did 4 of the 7 RIS. The other 3 RIS, like C/By mice, did not respond to PEA. This SDP is characteristic of response mediation by a single major dominant gene. However, conclusions must be tempered by the knowledge that the effect of only one dose of PEA was assessed and with only 7 RIS, the probability of obtaining such a bimodal SDP by chance is considerable.[3]

The BXD/Ty RIS Series

One of the best RIS models available for pharmacogenetic research is the BXD/Ty (Taylor) series derived from C57BL/6J (B6) and DBA/2J (D2) inbred mouse strains. Twenty-six BXD RIS are maintained, increasing the power of the model, and they have been inbred for well over 40 generations. To date, they have been typed for 171 genetic markers for the D2 or B6 type allele. The progenitor strains are known to differ genetically to a greater extent than most other commonly used inbred strains.[4] In addition, the progenitor strains have been compared extensively for drug sensitivity and preference, especially using alcohol, and have been found to differ greatly.[5,6,7,8,9,10,11]

Alcohol Acceptance

One example of use of the BXD RI series in a pharmacogenetic analysis is that of John Crabbe and his associates[9] in which the SDPs for various responses to ethanol (EtOH) were determined, the patterns analyzed for the presence of bimodal distributions, and the bimodally distributed SDPs compared to SDPs for known genetic markers. The SDPs of two of the characters examined, EtOH withdrawal severity and EtOH acceptance, provided evidence of major gene effects. The EtOH acceptance phenotype is particularly important because it has been shown to be genetically related to EtOH preference drinking and is, therefore, a possible measure of the reinforcing potency of EtOH.[12,13] Alcohol acceptance was further examined in a follow-up investigation which provides an excellent example of the use of RIS in genetic linkage analysis.[14] EtOH acceptance was measured in the B6 and D2 progenitor strains and in 15 of the RIS by measuring water intake in two consecutive 24-hour periods, fluid depriving the animals for 24 hours, and measuring 10% (v/v) EtOH intake in the next 24-hour period. Genetically variant proteins expressed in brain were identified in the same strains using 2-dimensional electrophoresis to screen for genetic variants in isoelectric point. Variants are inherited as co-dominants with F_1 animals showing 2 polypeptide spots of equal density and homozygous animals showing a dense spot for the acidic or basic allele. Results of these investigations mapped the putative genetic locus determining EtOH intake to a location at or near the LTW-4 gene on chromosome 1. Generally, strains exhibiting low EtOH intake, including the progenitor, D2, exhibited the acidic phenotype while high intake strains, including the B6 progenitor, exhibited the basic phenotype. These results were further corroborated in a separate experiment using a panel of 19 genetically diverse inbred mouse strains.[14] As pointed out by the authors, the imperfect correlation found between the LTW-4 type and alcohol acceptance magnitude could imply that (1) although one gene at or near the LTW-4 locus has a major influence on alcohol acceptance, other genes also modify this phenotype, (2) a gene linked to the LTW-4 locus mediates alcohol acceptance and infrequent cross-over has occurred between these loci, and (3) the relationship is not authentic, but is rather a random artifact produced by an imperfect methodology. However, these are still very exciting results since they suggest a molecular marker for a behavioral trait.

Genetic Determinants of Seizure Susceptibility

A great strength of inbred strain research, that extends equally to RIS, is that an individual of a given strain, tested at one time and location, is genetically identical to an individual of that strain tested at any other time and location, barring new mutations. Therefore, any number of data sets from a RIS battery can be compared or intercorrelated. For example, one common consequence of an extended period of alcohol use is physical dependence which can be indexed by seizure activity after alcohol withdrawal. In mice, one useful way of quantifying EtOH withdrawal severity is by determining handling-induced convulsion (HIC) severity over time.[15,16] Briefly, the withdrawing mouse is lifted by the tail, gently spun 180 degrees, and observed for seizure behavior. A rating scale is used to score seizure severity. Areas under the HIC curve from hours 0 to 15 after EtOH withdrawal were determined for 16 BXD RIS, D2, and B6 mice.[9] In another study of seizure sensitivity, 18 BXD RIS and their progenitor strains were tested for high pressure nervous syndrome (HPNS) Type I convulsion susceptibility.[17] Mice were exposed to compression in a heliox atmosphere until a convulsion was displayed. A bimodal SDP was observed, indicative of a major gene effect. Although these Type I convulsions pose a threat to deep-sea divers, of actual interest here are genetic determinants of susceptibility to seizures, whether induced by prolonged alcohol use or high pressure. Similar SDPs for HPNS seizure susceptibility and susceptibility to HICs after EtOH withdrawal might imply common genetic mediation of these seizure types. In fact, when the BXD RIS were classified as B6- or D2-like in their seizure responses, SDPs for the two seizure types differed for only 3 out of the 14 matched strains ($p = .029$, Binomial test). Strains with large HIC areas had lower convulsion threshold pressures, indicating greater relative susceptibility to seizures induced by both methods. Given this suggestion of genetic codetermination of two seemingly disparate seizure types, it would be especially pertinent to determine the genetic correlations among seizures occurring after withdrawal of a variety of drugs following dependence induction (e.g., EtOH, barbiturates, precipitated withdrawal after benzodiazepine abuse, etc.). Support for a genetic relationship between EtOH- and phenobarbital-withdrawal convulsions and between EtOH- and diazepam-withdrawal convulsions has been obtained using another genetic animal model.[18,19] Support for true genetic correlations would be considerably bolstered by positive data obtained with the RIS approach.

Genetic Vulnerability to Morphine Drinking

Horowitz et al.[20] and Horowitz[21] demonstrated that a normally avoided morphine sulfate in water solution (0.375 mg/ml) could be made highly preferred compared to tap water in some inbred strains of mice by the addition of saccharin. When morphine alone was given to 9 inbred mouse strains in a two-bottle *ad libitum* free choice situation (tap water vs. morphine solution), all but the C57BL/6A (Alberta) strain avoided the morphine solution, including the C57BL/6J (B6) and DBA/2J (D2) strains. Saccharin alone was highly preferred relative to tap water by all inbred strains except AKR/J, and the addition of 0.06% saccharin to the morphine solution, which presumably masked the bitter taste of morphine, caused a dramatic increase in morphine consumption in some strains, but no change in others. A very wide range of preference ratios resulted among the 9 inbred strains from a low of 4% (D2) to a high of 98% (B6) for the morphine-saccharin solution vs. tap water.[21] We know of no other drug, including EtOH, where the strain differences are more profound under a two-bottle (drug vs. water) choice situation. In the morphine-saccharin preferring B6 strain, daily consumption of morphine averaged

140 mg/kg. Under these conditions, some of the animals had fatal overdoses, and most of them exhibited diarrhea, a sign of morphine withdrawal, in response to challenge by an antagonist. In contrast, the D2 strain consumed less than 10 mg/kg per day under the same conditions, and showed no apparent drug effects. These workers also showed that the removal of the saccharin after 10 days of free choice morphine-saccharin led to only a moderate reduction in morphine consumption in the B6 strain. The morphine sulfate solution alone (0.375 mg/ml) continued to be preferred over tap water (75% preference ratio), indicating that the morphine itself can be preferred if consumption of morphine had been earlier enhanced by saccharin.[20] Saccharin alone was found to be highly preferred over tap water to a similar extent in both strains.

We have performed similar two-bottle choice experiments (morphine-saccharin vs. tap water vehicle) with B6 and D2 mice, and found that a gradual increase in morphine concentration resulted in a higher level of morphine consumption than did a fixed concentration in the drinking fluid.[7] After 14 days of two-bottle choice drinking, a high grade of physical dependence was demonstrable in B6 mice as shown by the elicitation of withdrawal signs (hypothermia, diarrhea, jumping, tremor, lacrimation), either with or without naloxone challenge. Given the dramatic differences between these 2 strains, we chose to perform similar studies in the BXD RIS to further elucidate the nature of the genetic influences. To the best of our knowledge, this is the first study involving opioids to utilize the BXD series.

Males from 20 of the BXD RIS were obtained from the Jackson Laboratory (Bar Harbor, ME) at 5-7 weeks of age and tested beginning at 8-12 weeks of age. The testing protocol was kept constant for all 20 strains (see below), with 5 strains run concurrently with an N of 7-8 for most strains. Under each condition listed below, one bottle contained the drug solution indicated and a second bottle contained only tap water. Thus, the mice were never forced to consume the drug solution. Both bottles were continuously present throughout the indicated periods. The position of the 2 bottles was alternated with each concentration change. Since it has been shown that B6 mice have a stronger preference for saccharin alone than do D2 mice,[7,22] it is possible that there may be palatability differences for the morphine-saccharin mixtures between the two strains. We sought to control for this by the use of quinine-saccharin mixtures, which would produce a similar aversive taste compared to morphine-saccharin mixtures, but would lack any opioid effects. We have previously shown that B6 and D2 mice do not differ in preference for quinine-saccharin solutions vs. tap water,[7] suggesting that the marked differences in morphine-saccharin consumption between these 2 strains are not due to palatability differences for sweetened alkaloid solutions. This approach was also used in the BXD strains reported below. Thus, palatability differences among the strains for saccharin-alkaloid solutions can be assessed and largely corrected for as a factor affecting morphine consumption. The protocol was as follows.

On Days:
Tap water alone was offered vs.:

1-5	0.2% saccharin (the maximally preferred conc. for B6 and D2)[7]
6-8	0.2% saccharin and 0.1 mg/ml quinine sulfate
9-12	0.2% saccharin and 0.2 mg/ml quinine sulfate
13-15	0.2% saccharin and 0.3 mg/ml quinine sulfate
16-19	0.2% saccharin and 0.4 mg/ml quinine sulfate
20-22	Tap water
23-26	0.2% saccharin and 0.3 mg/ml morphine sulfate
27-31	0.2% saccharin and 0.5 mg/ml morphine sulfate
32-36	0.2% saccharin and 0.7 mg/ml morphine sulfate
37-39	0.07% saccharin and 0.7 mg/ml morphine sulfate
40-43	0.02% saccharin and 0.7 mg/ml morphine sulfate

The results for the 20 BXD RIS and the 2 parental strains are shown in Table 1. All consumption values are for the last two days of each 3-4 day block, since this allowed the animals the maximum time possible to stabilize their consumption after the introduction of a new fluid. Consumption values given are averages of mg/kg consumed per day. The second column shows the saccharin consumption on Days 4 and 5 (last days of saccharin only presentation). The third column shows the quinine consumption on Days 18 and 19, the last days at the highest concentrations of quinine presented (0.4 mg/ml). For all strains but two, the highest consumption occurred at this concentration of quinine sulfate. The fourth column shows the morphine consumption on Days 34 and 35, the last days at the highest concentration of morphine presented (0.7 mg/ml). For all strains but one, the highest consumption occurred at this concentration of morphine sulfate. The fifth column shows the morphine consumption on the last days of saccharin withdrawal (Days 42 and 43), when the saccharin concentration was down to 1/10th of its earlier value. The complete withdrawal of saccharin was not performed due to an oversight. The sixth column shows the saccharin preference ratios on Days 4 and 5, which

Table 1. BXD RIS morphine two-bottle choice data. In order, columns 1-10 list: strain designation, saccharin (sac.) intake, quinine intake, high sac. (0.2%) morphine intake, low sac. (0.02%) morphine intake, sac. vs. water preference, quinine conc. reducing sac. preference below 50%, morphine conc. reducing sac. preference below 50%, morphine/quinine consumption ratio, and the standard error within-strain of the morphine/quinine ratio.

BXD STRAIN	<-----INTAKE IN mg/kg/day-----> SAC	QUININE	MORPHINE	LOWSAC	SAC PREF(%)	Q CONC <50%	M CONC <50%	M/Q RATIO	SE(M/Q)
12	475	11	97	31	77	0.23	0.63	12.20	3.85
22	264	9	96	35	61	0.15	0.73	10.12	1.70
B6	677	36	157	47	96	0.31	0.83	5.33	0.88
27	358	25	71	27	76	0.15	0.57	4.60	1.69
9	286	10	27	26	60	0.20	0.30	3.86	0.78
2	473	12	42	13	82	0.13	0.30	3.79	1.19
16	458	5	16	16	86	0.18	0.30	3.75	0.40
6	519	20	50	18	91	0.36	0.64	3.31	1.05
13	253	17	29	15	57	0.24	0.30	2.89	1.07
15	457	62	148	88	82	0.40	0.88	2.80	0.44
8	267	13	27	14	57	0.14	0.30	2.13	0.34
24	500	58	99	60	91	0.43	0.80	1.82	0.17
21	354	11	19	12	61	0.12	0.30	1.79	0.22
14	601	17	23	16	85	0.13	0.30	1.40	0.21
28	469	39	49	22	87	0.36	0.60	1.24	0.22
18	436	27	17	17	77	0.22	0.33	1.21	0.27
23	380	19	19	14	79	0.17	0.30	1.18	0.22
29	450	88	97	55	83	0.46	0.78	1.12	0.23
D2	294	24	16	20	59	0.23	0.30	0.64	0.08
1	332	32	16	21	74	0.25	0.38	0.63	0.12
5	1228	135	84	45	90	0.47	0.64	0.62	0.11
25	477	85	52	18	64	0.38	0.50	0.61	0.09
MEAN:	455	34	57	29	76	0.26	0.50	3.05	

represents the percentage of the total fluid intake (both bottles) consumed from the saccharin bottle. This represents another measure of the reinforcing effects of the saccharin alone, in addition to the consumption of saccharin measure shown in the second column. The seventh column shows the concentration of quinine necessary to reduce the preference ratio below 50%, i.e., when the animals consume less from the saccharin-quinine bottle than they do from the water bottle. This is an index of the ability of the saccharin (0.2%) to mask the bitter taste of quinine among the 22 strains. Mice failing to reduce their quinine-saccharin preference ratio below 50% at the highest concentration of quinine used (0.4 mg/kg) were arbitrarily given a value of 0.5 mg/ml. The eighth column shows the concentration of morphine necessary to reduce the preference ratio below 50%, in direct parallel with the previous measure with quinine. Mice failing to reduce their morphine-saccharin preference ratio below 50% at the highest concentration of morphine used (0.7 mg/ml) were arbitrarily given a value of 0.9 mg/ml.

The next to last column shows the ratio of morphine to quinine consumption (4th column/3rd column), which we believe is the best index of morphine drug-seeking behavior among those shown in the table. This ratio is valuable because it largely corrects for the palatability differences that appear to exist among the 22 strains for saccharin/alkaloid solutions on the presumption that morphine and quinine have similar bitter tastes. This is certainly true for humans, but more evidence is needed in the mouse. The morphine/quinine ratio also largely corrects for the presence of 0.2% saccharin, since it was coadministered with both alkaloids, and the amount of saccharin consumed was similar with either quinine or morphine administration. This amount was 170 vs. 162 mg/kg/day of saccharin, for the highest concentrations of quinine and morphine, respectively, over the entire data set. Looking at the two parental strains, B6 and D2, the former consumed over 10 times more morphine (in saccharin) than the latter (column 4), yet the consumption of quinine (also in saccharin) differed by only 1.5-fold between the 2 strains (column 3, $p < .01$). In an earlier study we found no differences in quinine (in saccharin) consumption between B6 and D2 strains.[7] In the present study, the morphine/quinine ratios were 5.3 for the B6 strain compared to 0.6 for the D2 strain. The strain difference in concentration of quinine needed to reduce quinine/saccharin preference below 50% versus water (column 7) was also relatively small (1.4-fold) compared to the morphine/quinine ratio (8.3-fold). Therefore, the two parental strains appear to differ to a relatively small extent in palatability of the saccharin-alkaloid solutions; thus most of the large strain difference in voluntary morphine consumption most plausibly reflects its postingestional effects.

Inspection of Table 1 reveals a number of interesting findings. A very large range of values are apparent among the 20 BXD and 2 parental strains for all of the variables. These large differences among strains are almost entirely genetically determined, since all of the strains were raised and tested under the same environmental conditions. This is in large measure due to the large differences seen between the two parental strains (B6 and D2), from which all of the BXD RIS were derived. In particular, the morphine/quinine ratios showed a very large range of values (over 40-fold) among the strains. For convenience, the BXD strains are listed in rank order from the highest to the lowest morphine/quinine ratios. BXD strains 12 and 22 showed ratios that resembled the B6 strain, with ratios greater than 5.0. Thus we can identify two BXD strains and the B6 strain as showing the highest morphine-seeking behavior with this protocol. In contrast, the last three BXD strains listed (1, 5 and 25) showed the lowest ratios (less than 0.5), and resembled the D2 parental strain in exhibiting the lowest morphine-seeking behavior under our voluntary consumption conditions. Consequently, the two extremes in voluntary morphine consumption are separated by at least a 10-fold difference in morphine-to-quinine consumption ratios. The other strains were roughly intermediate, with little or no suggestion of a bimodal distribution. Polygenic inheritance is therefore suggested, where no major gene effect for this phenotype can be identified.

It is interesting and important to note that the 2 BXD strains with the highest morphine-to-quinine ratios showed only average to below average consumption of saccharin, and preference for saccharin, compared to the other BXD strains. This is a reflection of the largely independent segregation of morphine/quinine ratios (column 9) from saccharin consumption (column 2) in the BXD series ($r = -.15$, n.s.). It is also of interest that one of the strains with an intermediate morphine-to-quinine ratio (BXD-15) had the highest consumption of morphine among the BXD strains. However, this strain also had the second highest consumption of quinine, which indicates that this strain may have a genetically determined taste deficit for bitter alkaloid compounds, leading to very high consumption of both alkaloids. The consumption of saccharin was only intermediate for this strain. Another interesting strain is BXD-5, which showed by far the highest consumption of saccharin of any of the BXD strains. This apparent "sweet tooth" in mice of this strain would be expected to lead to higher than average quinine and morphine consumption (both containing saccharin) for palatability reasons alone. This was certainly true for quinine, since this strain showed the highest quinine consumption of all strains tested; the consumption of morphine, however, was only somewhat above the mean for all 22 strains.

Table 2 shows the intercorrelations among the means of all measures taken with the two-bottle choice protocol in the 20 BXD and 2 parental strains. The magnitude of these correlation coefficients reflects the degree of commonality in genetic determination among any two of the 8 measures. Those correlations significantly different from zero are marked with an asterisk. Two findings are of interest here. First, the morphine/quinine ratios (variable 8) are not significantly correlated with any of the other consumption measures, showing that this measure of morphine seeking behavior does not appreciably overlap any of the other measures. Another finding of interest is that the various measures of morphine consumption show higher intercorrelations among themselves than they do with comparable indices of quinine consumption. Likewise, the various measures of quinine consumption show higher intercorrelations among themselves than they do with comparable measures of morphine consumption. These differences between the 2 alkaloids presumably reflect the important role of postingestional effects (e.g., psychoactive effects) regulating morphine intake, but not quinine intake, in the BXD RIS.

DISCUSSION AND CONCLUSIONS

As raised above, major gene effects are implied in a RIS analysis when a bimodal distribution of RIS values is obtained; when each mean RIS response resembles that of one of the progenitor strains. The work of Jeste et al.,[2] analyzing the effect of B-phenylethylamine on locomotor activity, provides an example of such an outcome. However, RI responses lying beyond the progenitor extremes, like those seen in our morphine consumption study (see column 9, Table 1), are a common finding with a plethora of possible explanations. There are two obvious and probable explanations. One is error of measurement. Given the variation in availability among the RIS, often requiring unequal and small sample sizes, outlier mean values are a likely outcome and response measurement validity may be an issue. Also in this category would be some undetected environmental difference that influenced the scores of particular strains during or prior to testing. The other highly probable reason for extreme RIS responses is a genetic one: polygenic mediation of the measured phenotype. In other words, this result could be attributable to a new combination of alleles in the extreme strain(s) not found in either of the progenitor

Table 2. Correlations among means of 20 BXD RIS and 2 progenitor strains for all consumption measures.

	1	2	3	4	5	6	7	8
1. Saccharin (0.2%) intake (mg/kg/day) vs. water	1.00							
2. Quinine intake (mg/kg/day) at highest quinine conc. (in 0.2% saccharin)	.70*	1.00						
3. Morphine intake (mg/kg/day) at highest morphine conc. (in 0.2% saccharin)	.36	.42	1.00					
4. Morphine intake (mg/kg/day) after saccharin withdrawal (to 0.02% saccharin)	.30	.54*	.85*	1.00				
5. Saccharin (0.2%) preference ratio vs. water (mls sac/ mls sac + mls water)	.65*	.34	.45	.39	1.00			
6. Quinine conc. (in 0.2% sac) yielding sac preference ratio < 50% vs. water	.52*	.83*	.53*	.65*	.46*	1.00		
7. Morphine conc. (in 0.2% sac) yielding sac preference ratio < 50% vs. water	.35	.51*	.93*	.84*	.51*	.70*	1.00	
8. Morphine/Quinine consumption ratio (Var 3/Var 2)	-.15	-.40	.41	.10	-.06	-.29	.30	1.00

* $p < .05$ for $r > 0$

strains. The progenitor responses may not define the extremes in attainable genetically-determined responses. Although no evidence for a major gene modulating morphine consumption was obtained with the BXD RIS analysis, this study was fruitful in identifying the response extremes for this behavior.

One less probable explanation for RIS responses more extreme than the progenitor strain responses might be the presence of a modifier gene which interacts epistatically with a specific allele at a relevant locus resulting in extremely high (or low) response values. For example, suppose a modifier gene modulates a "high morphine consumption" allele present in B6 mice, however, the dominant allelic form of this modifier is absent in the B6 and present in the D2 progenitor. Some of the RIs could have inherited both the dominant modifier and the B6 "high morphine consumption" allele resulting in morphine consumption values higher than those of the B6 progenitor. Another such explanation might be mutation at an important genetic locus resulting in a more extreme phenotype (e.g., saccharin consumption in BXD-5 mice). This explanation is especially unlikely when more than one RIS mean lies beyond a progenitor extreme, and even more unlikely when RIS values are obtained beyond both progenitor extremes.

Statistical evaluation of RIS data can be extremely problematic. The advocated method for determining modality is to apply analysis of variance (ANOVA) to the phenotypic data and, if a significant strain component is obtained, to follow up with appropriate multiple comparisons among means.[3] In this way, RIS may be classified as progenitor-like, as intermediate to the progenitors, or as more extreme than one of the progenitors (scoring higher than the high-scoring progenitor or lower than the low-scoring progenitor strain). However, this method is not often applied, rather, the "eyeball it" method is more commonly employed. An ANOVA is performed resulting in a significant strain difference and strain response means are compared to the progenitor means by visual appearance. Although this approach is not risky when the SDP appears to be continuous, when the pattern is visually bimodal the likelihood of making false conclusions about genetic linkage may be enhanced in the absence of more stringent statistical methods. This is especially true when the SDP is derived from a small number of strains. Given random fixation of all polymorphic alleles in the progenitor strains, the probability of observing a specific SDP is $(1/2)^k$, where k is the number of RIS tested, and the probability of not observing this SDP is 1 minus this value.[3] Therefore, the probability of observing a specific SDP is .008 for 7 strains, but only

.000001 for 20 strains. However, misclassification of even one strain could lead to choice of an incorrect linkage site when a large number of markers have been typed. On the other hand, given 26 RIS and 171 typed genetic markers, for the BXD RIS, the probability that one or more of the genetic marker SDPs will match a newly measured SDP is only .000003.[3] Thus, if two SDPs do match, the probability of genetic linkage is very high.

In conclusion, the existence of genetic factors determining sensitivity to drug effects, and modulating voluntary morphine drinking have been demonstrated using Recombinant Inbred mouse Strains. The morphine data suggest that genetic factors are important catalysts which may predispose certain individuals to abuse drugs. These data also indicate that identification of the specific gene products involved in determining vulnerability to morphine abuse will be complicated by the complexity of the genetic architecture underlying this trait. On the other hand, use of the RIS methodology has strongly implicated the involvement of a specific gene protein (or one produced by a closely linked gene) in determining alcohol acceptance, a trait closely related to alcohol preference drinking. This link was positively confirmed with a genetically diverse panel of inbred strains. There is compelling evidence for genetically-determined susceptibility to alcoholism in human populations[23] and it could be beneficial to determine if the rodent findings could be extrapolated to humans. In this age of explosive advances in molecular genetic techniques, identification of a gene involved in determining vulnerability to drug abuse could be the first step in the development of effective interventions.

REFERENCES

1. Bailey DW. Recombinant-inbred strains. Transplantation. 1971; 11:325-327.

2. Jeste DV, Stoff DM, Rawlings R, Wyatt RJ. Pharmacogenetics of phenylethylamine: Determination of heritability and genetic transmission of locomotor effects in recombinant inbred strains of mice. Psychopharmacology. 1984; 84:537-540.

3. Klein TW. Analysis of major gene effects using recombinant inbred strains and related congenic lines. Behav Genet. 1978; 8:261-268.

4. Taylor BA. Genetic relationship between inbred strains of mice. J Hered. 1972; 63:83-86.

5. Horowitz GP, Whitney G. Alcohol-induced conditioned aversion: Genotypic specificity in mice (Mus musculus). J Comp Physiol Psychol. 1975; 4:340-346.

6. Belknap JK, Belknap ND, Berg JH, Coleman R. Preabsorptive vs. post-

absorptive control of ethanol intake in C57BL/6J and DBA/2J mice. Behav Genet. 1977; 7:413-425.

7. Belknap JK. Physical dependence induced by the voluntary consumption of morphine in inbred mice. Pharmacol Biochem Behav. 1990; 35:311-315.

8. Tabakoff B, Kiianmaa K. Does tolerance develop to the activating, as well as the depressant, effects of ethanol? Pharmacol Biochem Behav. 1982; 17:1073-1076.

9. Crabbe JC, Kosobud A, Young ER, Janowsky JS. Polygenic and single-gene determination of responses to ethanol in BXD/Ty recombinant inbred mouse strains. Neurobehav Toxicol Teratol. 1983; 5:181-187.

10. Gwynn GJ, Domino EF. Genotype-dependent behavioral sensitivity to mu vs. kappa opiate agonists. I. Acute and chronic effects on mouse locomotor activity. J Pharmacol Exp Ther. 1984; 231:306-311.

11. Belknap JK, Noordewier N, Lamé M. Genetic dissociation of multiple morphine effects among C57BL/6J, DBA/2J and C3H/HeJ inbred mouse strains. Physiol Behav. 1989; 46:69-74.

12. Anderson SM, McClearn GE. Ethanol consumption: selective breeding in mice. Behav Genet. 1981; 11:291-301.

13. McClearn GE. The use of strain rank-orders in assessing equivalence of technique. Behav Methods Res Instrum. 1968; 1:49-51.

14. Goldman D, Lister RG, Crabbe JC. Mapping of a putative genetic locus determining ethanol intake in the mouse. Brain Res. 1987; 420:220-226.

15. Goldstein DB. Relationship of alcohol dose to intensity of withdrawal signs in mice. J Pharmacol Exp Ther. 1972; 180:203-213.

16. Kosobud A, Crabbe JC. Ethanol withdrawal in mice bred to be genetically prone or resistant to ethanol withdrawal seizures. J Pharmacol Exp Ther. 1986; 238:170-177.

17. McCall RD, Frierson D. A genetic analysis of susceptibility to the HPNS type I seizure in mice. In: Bachrach AJ, Matzen MM, eds. Undersea Physiology VII. Bethesda, MD: Undersea Med Soc., 1981:421-433.

18. Belknap JK, Danielson PW, Lamé M, Crabbe JC. Ethanol and barbiturate withdrawal convulsions are extensively codetermined in mice. Alcohol. 1988; 5:167-171.

19. Belknap JK, Crabbe JC, Laursen SE. Ethanol and diazepam withdrawal convulsions are extensively codetermined in WSP and WSR mice. Life Sci. 1989; 44:2075-2080.

20. Horowitz GP, Whitney G, Smith JC, Stephan FK. Morphine ingestion: Genetic control in mice. Psychopharmacology. 1977; 52:119-122.

21. Horowitz GP. Pharmacogenetic models and behavioral responses to opiates. In: McClearn GE, Deitrich RA, Erwin VG, eds. Development of Animal Models as Pharmacogenetic Tools, NIAAA Research Monograph No. 6. Washington D.C., U.S. Gov't printing office, 1981:209-232.

22. Fuller JL. Single locus control of saccharin preference in mice. J Hered. 1974; 65:33-36.

23. Goodwin DW. Alcoholism and heredity. Arch Gen Psychiatry. 1979; 36:57-61.

The Use of Recombinant Inbred Strains to Study Mechanisms of Drug Action

Jeanne M. Wehner, PhD
June I. Pounder, MS
Barbara J. Bowers, PhD

SUMMARY. Long-sleep (LS) and short-sleep (SS) mice which were selectively bred for sensitivity to the sedative-hypnotic effects of ethanol have been used extensively in the examination of sensitivity to ethanol as well as to other CNS depressants. Understanding the relationship between sensitivity to ethanol and other depressants using LS and SS mice has been limited to a two mouse line comparison because these mice do not exist as replicate lines. To circumvent this problem, DeFries et al.[5] have bred LSXSS recombinant inbred strains (LSXSS RIs) from a cross of LS and SS mice. These mice are being characterized on their responses to a variety of CNS depressants and agents that interact with the GABAergic system. Preliminary results are presented here on the sensitivity of these LSXSS RIs to pentobarbital, phenobarbital, and flurazepam as measured by sleep times. Additionally, analyses of seizure susceptibility to the GABAergic antagonist, bicuculline, in 24 LSXSS RIs indicate that there is no significant relationship between this measure of GABAergic function and sensitivity to ethanol as measured by the sleep-time response. These results are presented in the context of questions that can be resolved using RIs in drug-abuse research.

Jeanne M. Wehner is affiliated with the Institute for Behavioral Genetics and the School of Pharmacy; June I. Pounder is affiliated with the Institute for Behavioral Genetics; Barbara J. Bowers is affiliated with the Institute for Behavioral Genetics and the Department of Psychology, University of Colorado, Boulder, CO 80309.

Address correspondence to: Jeanne M. Wehner, Institute for Behavioral Genetics, Box 447, Boulder, CO 80309.

This work was supported by AA-03527 to JMW, a predoctoral traineeship to BJB, and BRSG funds to the University of Colorado from the Biomedical Research Support Grant Program, Division of Research Resources, NIH.

Several strategies are available to examine genetic and biochemical regulation of initial sensitivity to CNS depressants. These include surveys of inbred strains, heterogeneous stocks (HS) of rodents, selected lines of rodents and recombinant inbred strains. While each of these provides a powerful approach, large differences in drug sensitivity can most easily be observed after genetic selection of rodents that have been bred to produce animals that are either extremely resistant to a drug effect, or conversely extremely sensitive. Ideally, selection studies are performed in replicate so that two resistant, two sensitive and two control lines are available giving the researcher some power to correlate biochemical traits with behavioral sensitivities.[1]

A landmark study demonstrating the power of genetic selection was performed by McClearn and Kakihana.[2] In this study, animals differing in their initial sensitivity to the sedative-hypnotic effects of alcohol were produced. These lines were selected using the duration of loss of righting response as a measure of initial ethanol sensitivity. The long-sleep (LS) mice show a dramatically lengthened sleep time compared to the short-sleep (SS) mice, which are much less sensitive to an intraperitoneal injection of ethanol. Interestingly, LS and SS mice have been shown to differ in sensitivity to several other CNS depressants that like ethanol have the ability to produce physical dependence and therefore are candidates for drugs of abuse.[3,4] A problem arises in understanding whether the same genes regulate sensitivities to these various CNS depressants because LS and SS mice were not selected by an ideal design i.e., they do not exist in replicate. Therefore, the commonalities of sensitivity of LS and SS mice to benzodiazepines and some barbiturates might be the results of a fortuitous relationship not related to genes undergoing selection pressure, but rather the result of random genetic drift.

Recently, in order to circumvent these problems related to the LS/SS selection study, DeFries et al.[5] have bred 27 LSXSS recombinant inbred strains (LSXSS RIs). These strains were created by a systematic inbreeding of an F_3 cross of LS and SS mice. By this breeding strategy random or fortuitous linkages should be broken, allowing questions of common genetic and biochemical mechanisms to be addressed.[6] Some of these questions are discussed here and preliminary data on the LSXSS RIs are presented.

ARE RESPONSES TO CNS DEPRESSANTS REGULATED BY COMMON GENES?

We have begun to characterize these RIs at the Colorado Alcohol Research Center to understand whether responses to benzodiazepines, barbiturates and ethanol are mediated by common genes. LSXSS RIs provide a useful tool to sort out several controversies that have arisen in the drug abuse literature during the extensive use of the original LS and SS selected lines. For example, there has been considerable debate over the responses of LS and SS mice to barbiturates, especially pentobarbital. Erwin et al.[7] and later O'Connor et al.[8] reported that LS and SS mice did not differ in CNS sensitivity to pentobarbital. Although SS mice may sleep longer under pentobarbital than LS mice, O'Connor et al.[8] showed that this difference is due to drug metabolism rather than true CNS sensitivity differences because LS and SS mice regained the righting response at equal brain concentrations of pentobarbital. In contrast, McIntyre and Alpern reported that LS and SS mice were differentially responsive to pentobarbital and other CNS depressants as measured by sleep time[9,10] and promoted the idea that LS and SS mice were different in "tonic neural excitability."[11] The use of the LSXSS RIs should resolve this controversy by providing a more powerful technique than performing only a two line comparison with the original LS and SS mice.

Another benefit of the LSXSS RIs is that they afford the opportunity to study not only behavioral sensitivity, but also allow the examination of neural substrates regulating differential drug response via specific neurotransmitter systems. Because LS and SS mice have been shown to differ in several behaviors thought to be mediated by the GABAergic receptor system, recent emphasis has been placed on determining the relationship of these behavioral differences to biochemical differences in the GABAergic receptor complex. The GABA/benzodiazepine/barbiturate receptor complex is composed of several peptide subunits that have been isolated[12] and protein coding genes have been cloned.[13,14] This receptor complex contains binding sites for GABA; benzodiazepine agonists, antagonists, and inverse agonists; and barbiturates. These sites are coupled to a chloride ionophore. Heterogeneity of these binding sites and variation across brain regions has been demonstrated.[14] The functional nature of these heterogeneous subunits is unclear at this time, but a genetic approach using the LSXSS RIs might provide useful information to understand any functional correlates of the various receptor subunits.

GABA,[15] benzodiazepine,[16,17] and barbiturate receptors[15] have been characterized in LS and SS mice. No differences in receptor numbers or affinities were observed in these studies. However, the idea that LS and SS mice differ in the degree of coupling of the various subunits within the receptor complex is well supported. Ethanol potentiation of GABA stimulated Cl^- flux is greater in the more ethanol sensitive LS line[15] and a correlation between this potentiation and ethanol-induced sleep time in an HS stock of mice has been observed.[18] GABA enhancement of ^{3}H-flunitrazepam binding is greater in SS mice than in LS mice[17,19] and ethanol enhancement of BZ binding measured both *in vivo* and *in vitro* is greater in SS mice.[20,21] While it appears on the surface that this greater enhancement would be expected in the LS mice, it should be remembered that a greater number of genetic stocks e.g., the LSXSS RIs should be analyzed in order to understand these differences. With respect to benzodiazepine receptors, LS and SS mice have been shown to exhibit some degree of heterogeneity using heat denaturation experiments and beta-carboline competition.[16] Again, the functional relationship of this heterogeneity remains to be determined. LSXSS RIs may provide a tool to examine this functional relationship.

One purpose of the present research was to resolve controversial data regarding behavioral observations and to begin correlational studies of behavioral responses with neurochemical substrates in order to tease out common mechanisms regulating sensitivities to CNS depressants. The most important conclusion of the work thus far has been that generalities concerning common mechanisms are ill-founded in the face of recent data. LS and SS mice are not different in generalized CNS excitability, but rather behavioral commonalities depend very precisely on the dose of the drug used, the behavior measured, and on brain regional differences in GABAergic receptor parameters.

The data presented here are illustrative of the use of RIs to sort out some of these issues. Although data on all 27 RIs have not been compiled regarding drug sensitivities or behaviors of interest, we have measured several parameters in 8-26 of these strains. These data allow preliminary correlational analyses to be performed, but more complex strain distribution patterns, quantitative genetic analyses, or greater reliability in estimates of correlation will require the full complement of data on the LSXSS RIs.

To address the issue of genetic regulation of sensitivity to CNS depressants, sleep-time responses have been examined to sedative-hypnotic doses of ethanol, pentobarbital, phenobarbital, and the benzodiazepine, flurazepam. DeFries et al.[5] characterized the LSXSS RIs on a 4.1 g/kg 24% (w/v) dose of ethanol. They observed a distribution of sleep times in the LSXSS RIs with relatively few of the RIs responding like the LS mice. We have also characterized the LSXSS RIs using a 4.1 g/kg dose of ethanol, but using a lower concentration of ethanol, 20% (w/v) (Figure 1). We chose this dose and concentration because previous studies had shown a concentration dependency to ethanol-induced sleep times.[22] We have ob-

FIGURE 1

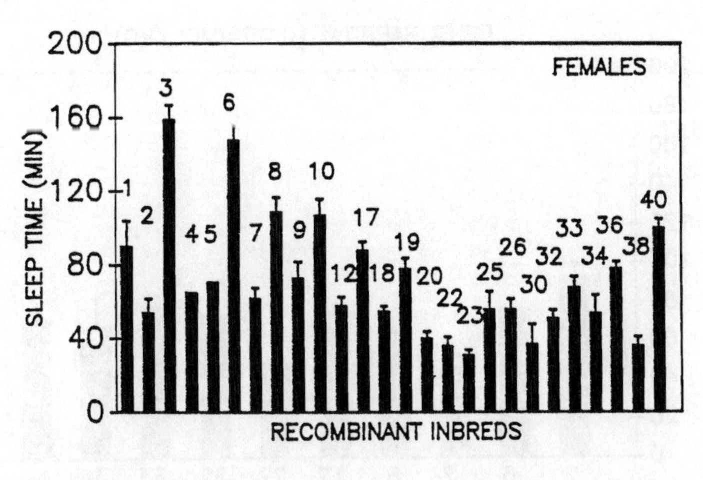

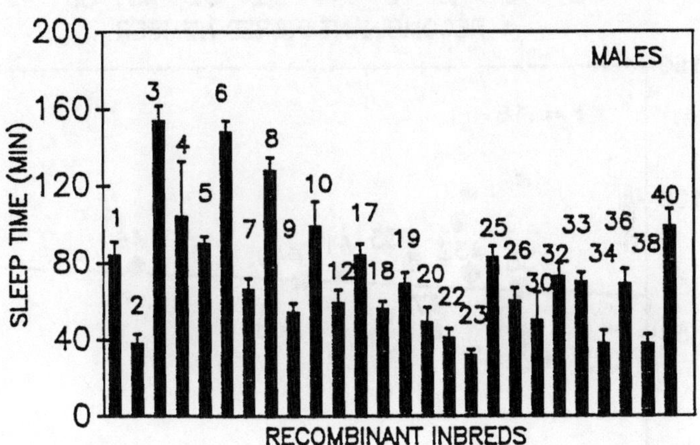

tained similar patterns of sleep-time scores in the RIs to those reported by DeFries et al.[5]

Pentobarbital-induced sleep time responses of female LSXSS RIs are shown in Figure 2. There are significant differences among the RIs in this response ($F(9, 59) = 3.67$, $P < .01$), but very importantly these differences do not correlate with differential ethanol sensitivity in the same strains ($r = 0.18$). These data suggest that there is no relationship between the sedative-hypnotic responses to two CNS depressants, ethanol and pentobarbital. The lack of commonality between the sedative-hyp-

FIGURE 2

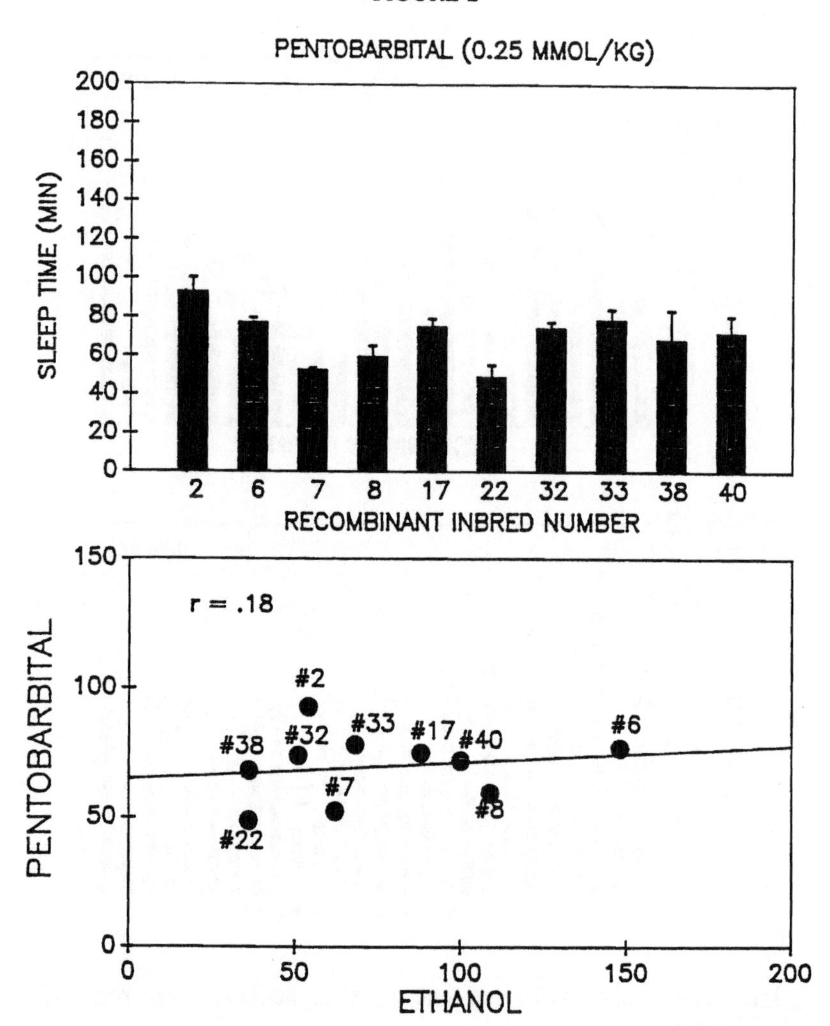

notic effects of ethanol and pentobarbital has also been demonstrated recently by Allan and Harris.[23] They used HS mice and assessed sleep-time to ethanol and then pentobarbital in several individual mice. The effects of ethanol and pentobarbital on muscimol-stimulated chloride flux were measured in these same mice. There was no significant correlation between ethanol sensitivity and pentobarbital sensitivity either as examined behaviorally or biochemically. Ethanol-induced sleep time was highly correlated with ethanol potentiation of muscimol-stimulated chloride flux. However, pentobarbital-induced sleep time did not correlate with ethanol-induced sleep time. Furthermore, pentobarbital potentiation of muscimol-stimulated Cl^- flux was not correlated with pentobarbital-induced sleep time response. Thus, although both ethanol and pentobarbital would be expected to potentiate GABA-stimulated Cl^- flux, there may be kinetic and/or mechanistic differences between the two drugs.

The sleep-time responses to phenobarbital (Figure 3) vary significantly across the LSXSS RIs tested ($F(8,53) = 3.10$ $P < .01$) and correlate with ethanol-induced sleep time responses ($r = .62$, $P < .01$). The fact that pentobarbital and phenobarbital are different is interesting. While other barbiturates remain to be tested, we hypothesize at this point in the research that the lipid solubility of barbiturates may be important in determining the degree of sensitivity in the RIs. Marley et al.[3] tested 19 depressants including alcohols and barbiturates that vary in lipid solubility in LS and SS mice for differential CNS sensitivity as measured by sleep time. A negative correlation was observed between the degree of lipid solubility i.e., the octanol-water partition coefficient, and the sleep-time differential between LS and SS mice. Their data indicated that LS and SS mice differ more radically in CNS sensitivity to agents that have water solubilities resembling ethanol. They hypothesized that common genes regulating some membrane parameters that differentiate lipid- and water-soluble agents may have been fixed during the selection process. Additional support for this hypothesis awaits testing many more LSXSS RIs with other barbiturates and alcohols differing in lipid solubility.

Marley et al.[4] demonstrated that LS mice were more sensitive to the sedative hypnotic effects of benzodiazepines as measured by flurazepam-induced sleep time. McIntyre and Alpern[9] showed differential sensitivity with chlordiazepoxide. Figure 4 shows the sleep-time response of several LSXSS RIs to the benzodiazepine, flurazepam. There are significant train differences ($F(7,37) = 12.19$, $P < .001$) and a positive significant correlation with ethanol-induced sleep time ($r = .82$, $P < .01$). These data suggest that response to this benzodiazepine may share some commonality with sensitivity to high-dose effects of ethanol. This study provides an independent confirmation of the work of Allan and Harris[22] showing a positive and significant correlation between ethanol-induced sleep time and flunitrazepam potentiation of muscimol-stimulated Cl^- flux in HS mice. Neither our work, nor that of Allan and Harris,[23] supports common-

FIGURE 3

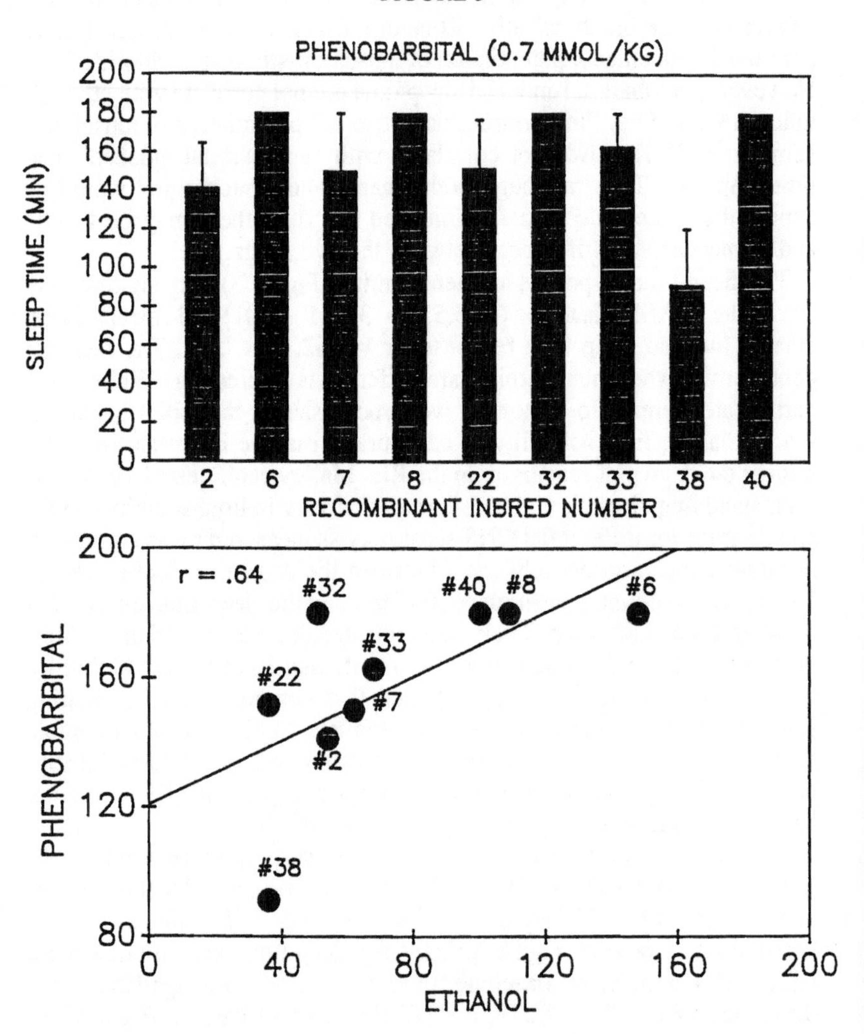

ality between pentobarbital and flurazepam because no correlation was observed between sleep-time responses between the two agents (r = .04).

The fact that there is some commonality between flunitrazepam and ethanol sensitivity when sleep time is the measure should not be generalized to all responses. Our previous studies showed that while LS mice

FIGURE 4

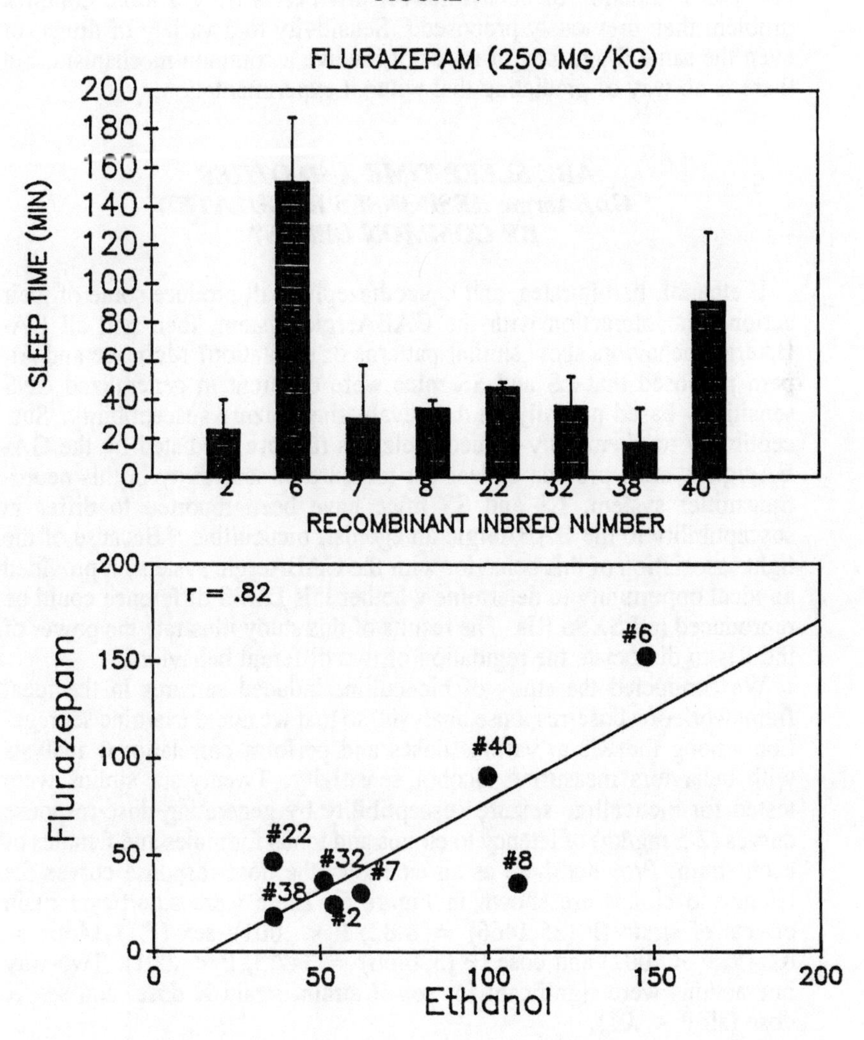

were more sensitive on this measure, SS mice were more sensitive to the lower dose anticonvulsant effects of flurazepam.[4] Moreover, flurazepam-induced hypothermia shows no differential response between LS and SS mice. The anxiolytic response of LS mice to another benzodiazepine, diazepam, was greater than that of SS mice.[24] These contrasting data indicate that evaluation of behavioral sensitivities is truly a more complex problem than previously proposed.[11] Sensitivity to a variety of drugs, or even the same drug, may or may not involve a common mechanism, but there is no way of predicting that without experimentation.

ARE SLEEP TIME AND OTHER GABAergic RESPONSES REGULATED BY COMMON GENES?

If ethanol, barbiturates, and benzodiazepines all produce some of their actions via interaction with the GABAergic system, then will all GABAergic behaviors show similar patterns of regulation? McIntyre and Alpern proposed that LS and SS mice were different in generalized CNS sensitivity based partially on data evaluating seizure susceptibility. Susceptibility to chemically-induced seizures that are mediated by the GABAergic system provide a clear-cut measure of sensitivity in this neurotransmitter system. LS and SS mice have been reported to differ in susceptibility to the GABAergic antagonist, bicuculline.[25] Because of the tight association of this behavior with the GABAergic system, it provided an ideal opportunity to determine whether this LS/SS difference could be reproduced in LSXSS RIs. The results of this study illustrate the power of the RIs to dissociate the regulation of two different behaviors.

We conducted the study of bicuculline-induced seizures in the ideal framework of a dose-response analysis, so that we could examine segregation among the RIs at various doses and perform correlational analysis with behaviors measuring alcohol sensitivity. Twenty-six strains were tested for bicuculline seizure susceptibility by generating dose-response curves (2-5 mg/kg) of latency to clonus and tonus for males and females of each strain. Provided here as an example, the dose-response curves for latency to clonus are shown in Figure 5. There were significant main effects of strain ($F(25,1466) = 8.82$, $P < .001$); sex ($F(1,1466) = 82.45$, $P < .001$) and dose ($F(3,1466) = 347.3$, $P < .001$). Two-way interactions were significant for sex X strain, strain X dose, and sex X dose (all $P < .01$).

Frequency histograms that show the number of RIs responding at various levels of seizure susceptibility are shown in Figures 6 and 7 by dividing latencies into periods of one-hundred seconds. These histograms indicate that there is not a bimodal distribution indicative of a single gene effect. Although the binding of bicuculline might *a priori* seem like an event that might be regulated by binding directly at the GABA subunit of the receptor complex, other genes such as those regulating seizure initia-

FIGURE 5

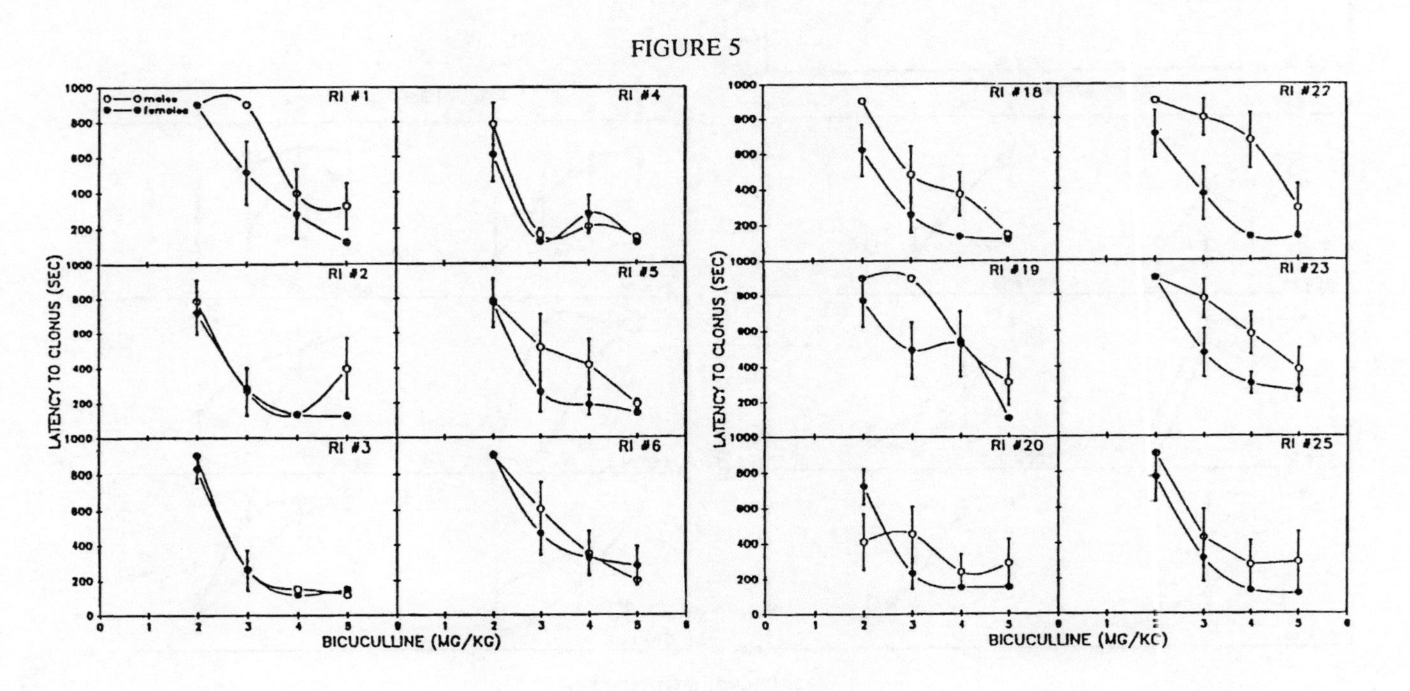
males
females
RI #1
RI #2
RI #3
RI #4
RI #5
RI #6
RI #18
RI #19
RI #20
RI #22
RI #23
RI #25
LATENCY TO CLONUS (SEC)
BICUCULLINE (MG/KG)
BICUCULLINE (MG/KC)

FIGURE 5 (continued)

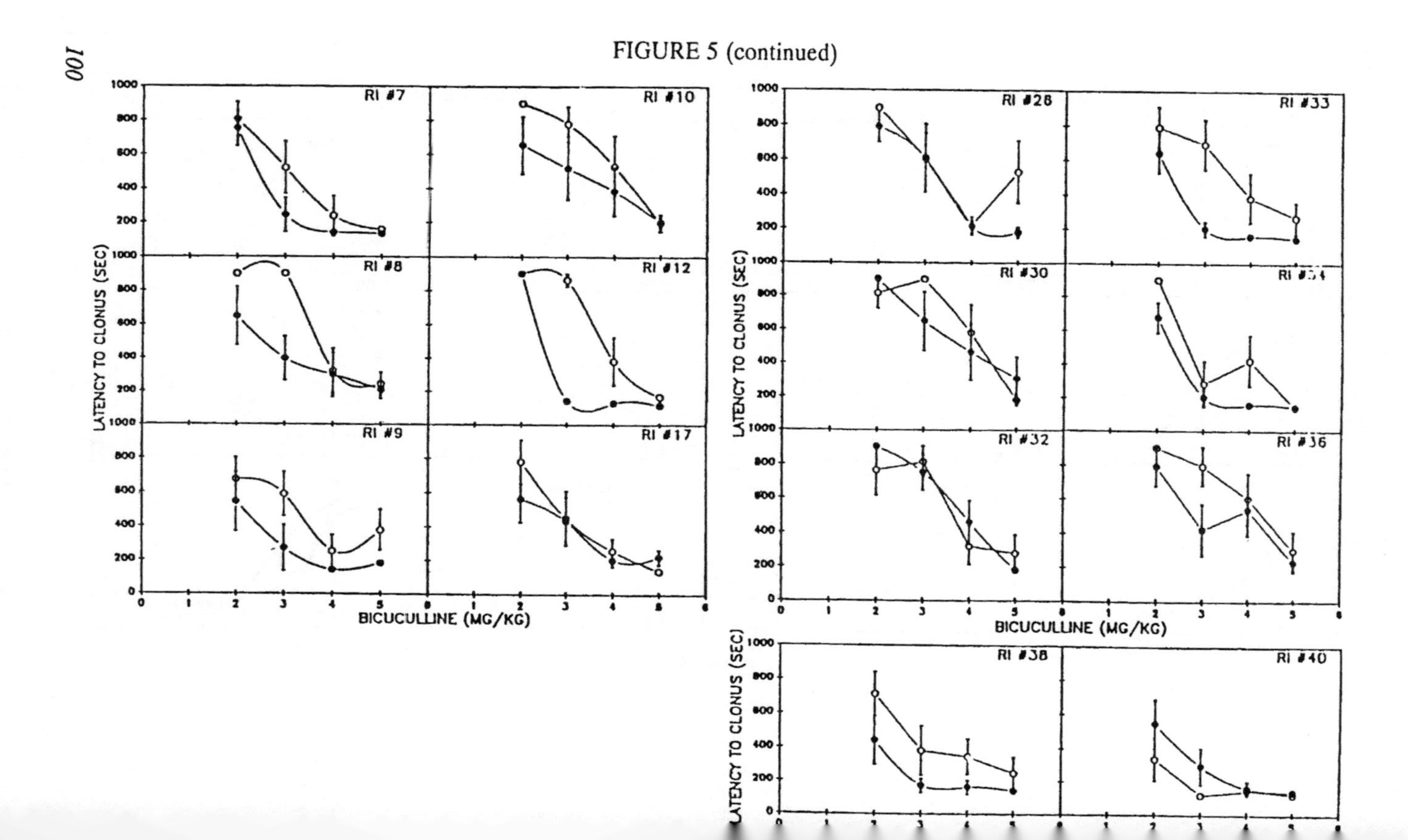

FIGURE 6

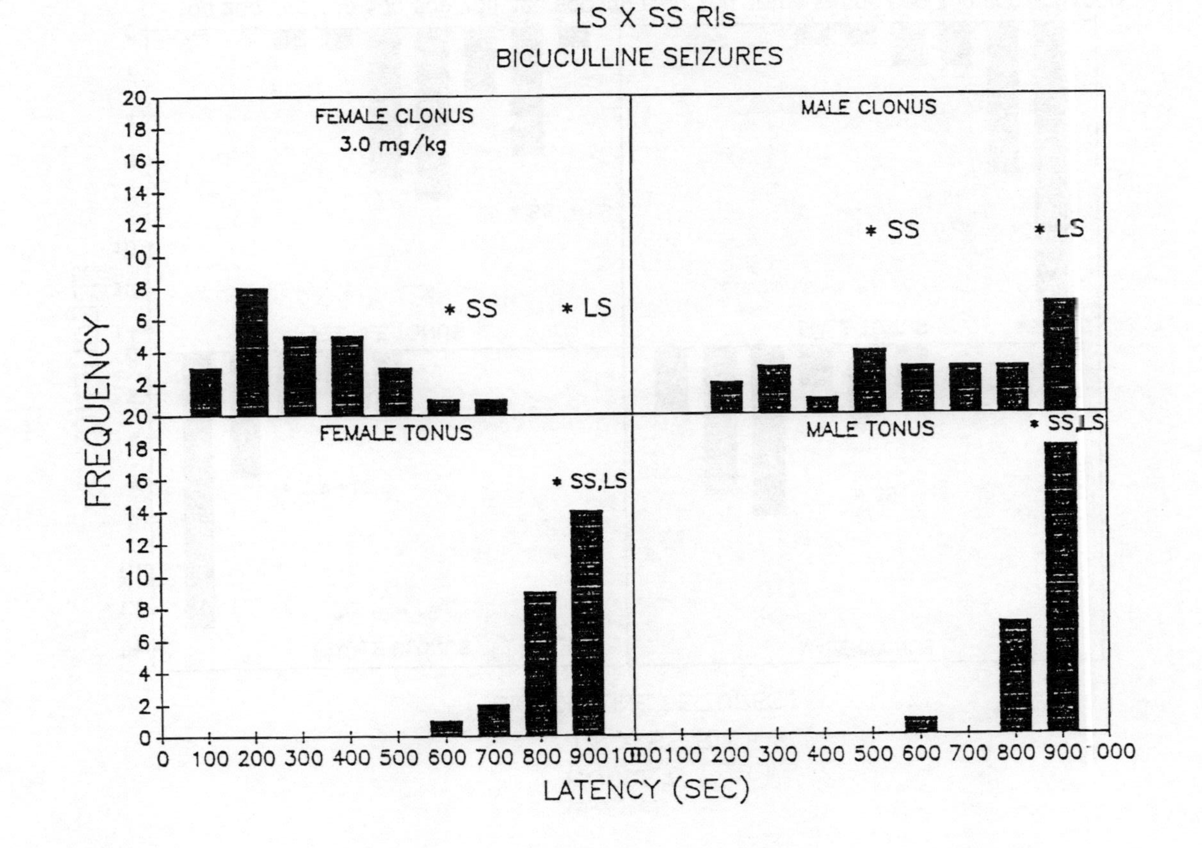

LS X SS RIs
BICUCULLINE SEIZURES
FEMALE CLONUS
3.0 mg/kg
* SS
* LS
MALE CLONUS
* SS
* LS
FEMALE TONUS
* SS,LS
MALE TONUS
* SS,LS
FREQUENCY
LATENCY (SEC)
0
2
4
6
8
10
12
14
16
18
20
100
200
300
400
500
600
700
800
900

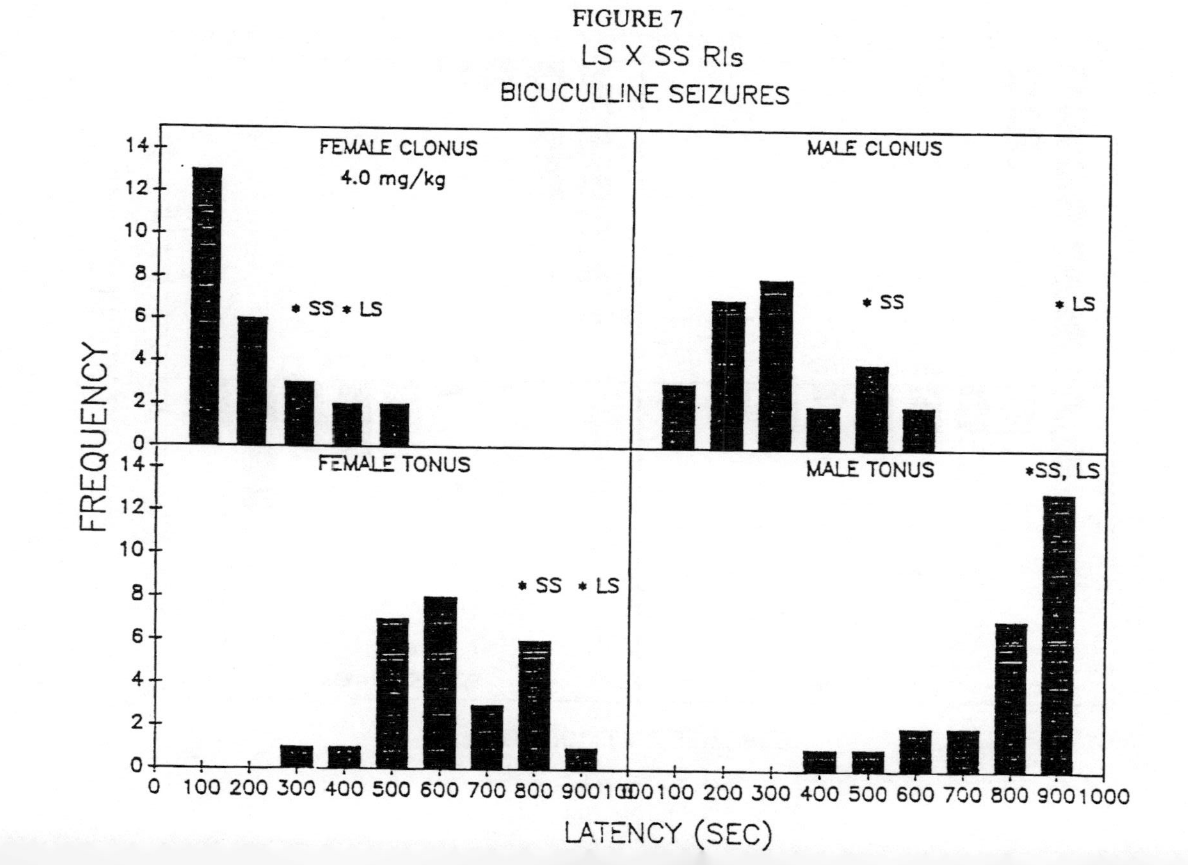

FIGURE 7
LS X SS RIs
BICUCULLINE SEIZURES

tion and propagation are undoubtably involved and lead to a more complex pattern of response.

Correlational analyses were performed with seizure latency scores at clonus and tonus at the 3.0 mg/kg or 4.0 mg/kg bicuculline dose with ethanol-induced sleep time in the RIs. These correlations are summarized in Table 1. In no comparison was the correlation significant. These seizure data indicate that there is a dissociation between seizure susceptibility to bicuculline and sensitivity to ethanol-induced sleep times. Although LS and SS mice may differ on this measure, this difference appears to be a fortuitous relationship. Thus, susceptibility to GABAergic seizures and ethanol-induced hypnosis are not regulated by common genes. Furthermore, this lack of commonality suggests that seizure susceptibility may be regulated by GABA receptors distinctly different from those regulating the actions of ethanol on the chloride ionophore. Simply stated, not all GABAergic responses are regulated by common genes. This conclusion is supported by recent cloning studies of the GABA/benzodiazepine receptor

TABLE 1. Correlations estimated from LSXSS RI Strain Means. Ethanol-induced Sleep Times

Bicuculline Seizures			
3.0 mg/kg			
latency to clonus,	females	0.04	n.s.
	males	-0.09	n.s.
latency to tonus,	females	-0.05	n.s.
	males	-0.01	n.s.
4.0 mg/kg			
latency to clonus,	females	0.06	n.s.
	males	-0.30	n.s.
latency to tonus,	females	0.07	n.s.
	males	0.04	n.s.

complex in which multiple genes have been cloned for the respective subunits.[13]

Recently, Peris et al.[25] have provided additional support for this dissociation using receptor autoradiographic techniques. They observed that the amount of binding of the cage convulsant ^{35}S-TBPS, which is thought to bind the chloride ionophore, was different in the superior and inferior colliculi of LS and SS mice. Examination of this difference in LSXSS RIs indicated that the amount of binding in these regions was significantly correlated with susceptibility to bicuculline-induced seizures, but not with ethanol-induced sleep time. These results provide a potential neural substrate underlying differential seizure susceptibility to bicuculline and again point to the fact that heterogeneity of GABAergic receptors across brain regions may be important for functional differences.

The seizure data presented here as well as those reported by Marley and Wehner[26] using an alternate GABAergic seizure producing agent, 3-mercaptopropionic acid (3MP), an inhibitor of GABA formation, reiterate the idea that generalized CNS excitability is not different in LS and SS mice. In this previous study, it was shown that LS mice are more susceptible to 3-mercaptopropionic acid seizures than are SS mice. Again, these data show that specificity of response will depend precisely on the agent used e.g., the actions of a presynaptic agent such as the GAD inhibitor, 3-MP, differs from the antagonist, bicuculline, which presumably is binding at a postsynaptic site.

LIMITATIONS OF THE RECOMBINANT INBRED STRAIN APPROACH

As with any approach, there are some limitations to the use of RIs to resolve questions of differential sensitivity to drugs and the neural substrates regulating these sensitivities. Importantly, unless the behavioral sensitivity is regulated by a single gene, one must resort to correlational analysis. In order to provide the most reliable estimate of genetic correlations, a large number of strains must be examined and sometimes that is prohibitively expensive. How does one resolve this problem? Probably the best solution is to put any correlational data in the context of information derived from studies performed by a different method. As an example, the pentobarbital data presented above were discussed in the context of data derived from the HS study of Allan and Harris.[23] The data from our study and theirs support the same conclusion and therefore add credibility to the assumption that ethanol- and pentobarbital-induced sleep-time are not regulated by same genes. In the absence of such supporting information, conclusions from correlational data should be viewed as tentative.

Another problem can be in the assessment of what inbreeding means in the context of newly derived RIs such as the LSXSS RIs. These newly derived strains should theoretically after 20 generations of inbreeding reach homozygosity at all loci. However, in actual fact, 20 generations of inbreeding may not be sufficient. For example, DeFries et al.[5] discuss the segregation of the c-locus (albinism) in the LSXSS RIs. Even after 25 generations of inbreeding, one of the LSXSS RIs is not fixed at this locus resulting in a mixture of coat colors in this strain. Any correlation that is influenced to a great degree by the inclusion of this strain should be considered very tentative until many other strains can be included.

In addition, a difficult question concerning environmental interactions arises when using RIs because they are inbred strains. The assumption is usually made that if all inbred strains in a study are treated alike and the environment tightly controlled, then correlations derived from population means should approximate genetic correlations.[27] However, if a particular strain responds differentially to a particular environmental stimulus (GXE interaction) then the population mean will be influenced and the overall correlation less reliable. Again, the impact of this environmental influence, and occurrence of chance associations between two traits can be limited by the use of a large number of strains. Lastly, as stressed by Crabbe,[28] variability in sensitivity among the RIs is limited to that of the original parental stocks. A comparison across several other inbred strains is essential to generalize to sensitivity in mice in general.

Although RI data are unquestionably more powerful than data from a single outbred stock of rodent, or a two selected line or strain comparison, it should always be kept in mind that correlational data does not prove causality and that testing a large number of strains is always the best application of the RI methodology.

In summary, the LSXSS RIs provide a valuable tool to assess mechanisms that may underlie sensitivity to CNS depressants, and to investigate the association of these behavioral traits with neural substrates. The use of this pharmacogenetic tool in the field of drug abuse should provide a novel approach to complement traditional studies of ethanol, benzodiazepines, and barbiturates.

REFERENCES

1. DeFries JC. Selective breeding for behavioral and pharmacological responses in laboratory mice. In: Gershon ES, Mattysse S, Breakfield XO, Ciaranello RD. Genetic Research Strategies for Psychobiology and Psychiatry. 1981: 199-213.

2. McClearn GE, Kakihana K. Selective breeding for ethanol sensitivity: SS

and LS mice. In: McClearn GE, Deitrich RA, Erwin VG, eds. Development of animal models as pharmacogenetic tools. United States Government Printing Office, Washington, D.C., 1981: 147-159.

3. Marley RJ, Miner LL, Wehner JM, Collins AC. Differential effects of central nervous system depressants in long-sleep and short-sleep mice. Journ. Pharmacol. Exper. Ther. 1986; 238: 1028-1033.

4. Marley RJ, Freund RK, Wehner JM. Differential response to flurazepam in long-sleep and short-sleep mice. Pharmacol. Biochem. Behav. 1988; 31: 453-458.

5. DeFries JC, Wilson JR, Erwin VG, Petersen DR. LSXSS REcombinant inbred strains of mice: Initial characterization. Alcoholism: Clin. Exper. Res. 1989; 13: 196-200.

6. Baily DW. Recombinant-Inbred Strains: An aid to finding identity, linkages, and function of histocompatibility and other genes. Transplantation 1971; 11: 325-327.

7. Erwin VG, Heston WDW, McClearn GE, Deitrich RA. Effects of hypnotics on mice genetically selected for sensitivity to ethanol. Pharmacol. Biochem. Behav. 1976; 4: 679-683.

8. O'Connor MF, Howerton TC, Collins AC. Effects of pentobarbital in mice selectively bred for differential sensitivity to ethanol. Pharmacol. Biochem. Behav. 1982; 17: 245-248.

9. Alpern H, McIntyre TD. Evidence that the selectively-bred long-sleep and short-sleep mouse lines display common narcotic reactions to many depressants. Psychopharmacol. (Berlin); 1985; 85: 456-459.

10. McIntyre TD, Alpern HP. Thiopental, phenobarbital, and chlordiazepoxide induce the same differences in narcotic reaction as ethanol in long-sleep short-sleep selectively bred mice. Pharmacol. Biochem. Behav. 1986; 24: 895-898.

11. McIntyre TD, Alpern HP. Reinterpretation of the literature indicates differential sensitivities of long-sleep and short-sleep mice are not specific to alcohol. Psychopharmacol. 1985; 87: 379-389.

12. Stephenson FA. Understanding the $GABA_A$ receptor: A chemically gated ion channel. Biochem. J. 1988; 249: 21-32.

13. Schofield PR, Darlison MG, Fujita N, Burt DR, Stephenson FA, Rodriguez H, Rhee LM, Ramachandran J, Reale V, Glencorse TA, Seeburg PH, Barnard EA. Sequence and functional expression of the $GABA_A$ receptor shows a ligand-gated receptor super-family. Nature 1987; 328: 221-227.

14. Levitan ES, Schofield PR, Burt DR, Rhee LM, Wisden W, Kohler M, Fujita N, Rodriquez HF, Stephenson A, Darlison MG, Barnard EA, Seeburg PH. Structural and functional basis for $GABA_A$ receptor heterogeneity. Nature 1988; 335: 76-79.

15. Allan AM, Harris RA. Gamma-aminobutyric acid and alcohol actions: Neurochemical studies of long-sleep and short-sleep mice. Life Sciences 1986; 39: 2005-2015.

16. Marley RJ, Stinchcomb A, Wehner JM. Further characterization of benzodiazepine receptor differences in long-sleep and short-sleep mice. Life Sciences 1988; 43: 1223-1231.

17. Marley RJ, Wehner JM. GABA enhancement of flunitrazepam binding in mice selectively bred for differential sensitivity to ethanol. Alcohol and Drug Research 1986; 7: 25-32.

18. Allan AM, Spuhler KP, Harris RA. Gamma-aminobutyric acid activated chloride channels: relationship to genetic differences in ethanol sensitivity. Journ. Pharmacol. Exper. Ther. 1988; 244: 866-870.

19. McIntyre TD, Trullis R, Skolnick P. Differences in the biophysical properties of benzodiazepine/gamma-aminobutyric acid receptor chloride channel complex in long-sleep and short-sleep mouse lines. Journ. Neurochem. 1988; 51: 642-647.

20. Miller LG, Greenblatt DJ, Barnhill JG, Shader RI. Differential modulation of benzodiazepine receptor binding by ethanol in LS and SS mice. Pharm. Biochem. Behav. 1988; 29: 471-477.

21. Bowers BJ, Wehner JM. Interaction of ethanol and stress with the GABA/BZ receptor in LS and SS mice. Brain Res. Bull. 1989; 23: 53-59.

22. Gilliam DM, Collins AC. Concentration-dependent effects of ethanol in long-sleep and short-sleep mice. Alcoholism: Clin. Exp. Res. 1983, 7: 337-342.

23. Allan AM, Harris RA. Sensitivity to ethanol hypnosis and modulation of chloride channels does not cosegregate with pentobarbital sensitivity in HS mice. Alcoholism: Clin. Exp. Res. 1989; 13: 428-434.

24. Stinchcomb A, Bowers BJ, Wehner JM. The effects of ethanol and RO 15-4513 on elevated plus-maze and rotarod performance in long-sleep and short-sleep mice. Alcohol 1989; 6: 369-376.

25. Phillips TJ, Dudek BC. Bicuculline-induced seizures in mice which differ in sensitivity to ethanol. Neuroscience Abstracts 1983; 9: 1240.

26. Peris J, Wehner JM, Zahniser NR. [^{35}]TBPS binding sites are decreased in colliculi of mice with a greater predisposition to bicuculline induced seizures. Brain Res. 1989; 503: 288-295.

27. Hegman JP, Possidente B. Estimating genetic correlations from inbred strains. Behav. Genetics 1981; 11: 103-114.

28. Crabbe JC. Genetic animal models in the study of alcoholism. Alcoholism: Clin. Exp. Res. 1989; 13: 120-127.

Progress Towards the Development of Animal Models of Smoking-Related Behaviors

Allan C. Collins, PhD
Michael J. Marks, PhD

SUMMARY. Human twin studies have indicated that genetic factors influence whether people do, or do not, smoke and may also influence amount of tobacco used. Studies in the authors' laboratory have demonstrated that inbred mouse strains differ in sensitivity to many actions of a first challenge dose of nicotine These strain differences are due, in part, to differences in the number of brain nicotinic receptors. Mouse strains also differ in the development of tolerance to nicotine and subtle differences in chronic nicotine-induced increases in the number of brain nicotinic receptors have been detected. Preliminary data suggest that mouse strains differ in oral self-selection of nicotine containing solutions which may suggest genetic influences on rewarding effects on nicotine. These results suggest that humans may also differ, for genetic reasons, in sensitivity to nicotine, in the development of tolerance to nicotine and in rewarding effects of nicotine. Presumably, those individuals who are resistant to nicotine's toxic actions and sensitive to its rewarding

---

Allan C. Collins is affiliated with the Institute for Behavioral Genetics, Department of Psychology, and School of Pharmacy, and Michael J. Marks is affiliated with the Institute for Behavioral Genetics and School of Pharmacy, University of Colorado, Boulder, CO 80309.

The authors wish to thank Steven Campbell, Elena Romm and Scott Robinson for technical assistance and Kari Zempel for assistance in preparation of the manuscript.

Reprint requests may be obtained from Allan C. Collins, Institute for Behavioral Genetics, Campus Box 447, University of Colorado, Boulder, CO 80309.

This work was supported by DA-03194 and DA-05131. A.C.C. is supported, in part, by a Research Scientist Development Award from the National Institute on Drug Abuse (DA-00116).

effects are more likely to become smokers if tobacco experimentation is initiated.

The issue of why a given individual does, or does not, use a psychoactive substance is a complex one. For illicit drugs, such as cocaine or the opiates, many individuals will not use these agents because environmental factors will limit availability, and or desirability. Obviously, a given individual, no matter what his or her biology may be, will not become dependent on a given drug if the drug is not available in that individual's environment. Similarly, some individuals will not use a substance, even if it is readily available, if factors in that individual's environment preclude or antagonize experimentation.

The use of tobacco products is not restricted, for most people, by issues such as legality; tobacco is readily available. Despite this ready availability, not everyone experiments with tobacco and not everyone who does so becomes a devoted user. Certainly there are environmental factors that contribute to this. Attitudes such as "smoking is sophisticated" certainly promote use whereas concerns about health effects of smoking probably decrease use. In addition, it seems likely that biological factors contribute to whether people do or do not use tobacco. Over 30 years ago, Fisher[1,2] reported that concordance for smoking behavior was greater in monozygotic (MZ, identical) twins than was concordance in dizygotic (DZ, fraternal) twins. The twins were listed as concordant if both members of the twin pair were smokers or non-smokers. Fisher's studies included twins that were reared together and twins that were reared apart; rearing status did not affect the concordance. These data indicated that genetic factors are important in regulating smoking behavior. Several subsequent studies have replicated Fisher's findings[3-7] (see Table 1 for the results of these studies). One of these studies,[4] analyzed the smoking habits of Danish MZ and DZ twins in greater depth. The twins were divided into non-smokers, occasional smokers, former smokers, regular smokers and heavy smokers and, for smokers, the type of tobacco (cigar, pipe, cigarette) used was assessed. Concordance was greater for MZ twins than for DZ twins not only for smoking status but also for amount and type of tobacco used.

The finding that concordance for tobacco use is greater in MZ twins than in DZ twins indicates that genetic factors influence smoking behavior. Genetic factors could promote tobacco use or, alternatively, genetic factors could inhibit tobacco use. Unfortunately, none of the twin studies of smoking behavior have shed any light on whether genetic factors promote or inhibit tobacco use nor do these studies suggest what factors might be inherited that would influence tobacco use. Our research group has been

TABLE 1. Genetics of Human Tobacco Use

Study	Subjects	Sex	Rearing	Concordance MZ	Concordance DZ
Fisher, 1958a[1]	German	M	---	39/51	11/31
Fisher, 1958b[2]	German	F	total	44/53	9/13
			together	21/26	
			apart	23/27	
Friberg et.al.,[3] 1959	Swedes	MF	---	45/59	34/59
Raaschou-Nielsen,[4] 1960	Danes	M	---	106/147	131/223
		F	---	141/196	190/328
Shields, 1962[5]	English	-	together	30/42	10/20
		-	apart	33/42	---
Conterio & Chiarelli, 1962[6]	Italian	M	---	31/34	28/43
Pedersen, 1981[7]	Swedes	MF	---	59/75	38/62

In each of the studies cited above, monozygotic (MZ) and dizygotic (DZ) twins were questioned regarding their smoking behaviors. The twins were judged to be concordant if both members of a twin pair were either smokers or non-smokers. The difference in the concordance ratio (# of twin pairs who are concordant divided by total # of twin pairs studied) for MZ twins versus DZ twins is an estimate of the genetic influence on smoking behavior.

attempting to identify potential factors that would promote or limit tobacco use by studying the responses of mice to nicotine, the most potent psychoactive agent in tobacco. Nicotine is being studied, rather than tobacco itself, because smokers seem to alter puff rate and depth of inhalation to carefully titrate blood nicotine levels[8,9] and administration of mecamlylamine, a potent inhibitor of brain nicotinic receptors, results in altered (increased) smoking, probably in an attempt to overcome the receptor blockade.[10,11]

Our studies have focused, until very recently, on ascertaining whether genetic factors influence initial sensitivity to nicotine (sensitivity to the first dose of nicotine) and whether genetic factors regulate tolerance development. The initial sensitivity experiments have measured a variety of responses to nicotine that we suspect are more related to why people would choose not to smoke rather than why they would choose to smoke. The rationale for our studies is that it may be that individuals who are very sensitive to nicotine's noxious effects (tremor, nausea, change in heart rate and blood pressure) will choose not to smoke, unless they develop tolerance to these debilitating effects of nicotine. We have chosen to ascertain whether genetic factors influence initial sensitivity to nicotine by studying nicotine responses in inbred mouse strains. The mouse was used because a wide variety of inbred strains are available thereby increasing the probability that genetically-induced variation will be found. Inbred strains, which are like human MZ twins in that all members of a strain are genetically identical to all other members, were used because repeated testing on individuals can be avoided. The "n" can be increased by testing additional animals from the strain.

INITIAL SENSITIVITY TESTS

Nicotine elicits a wide variety of effects and both stimulant and depressant effects have often been reported. For example, in their 1889 report on nicotine effects in autonomic ganglia, Langley and Dickinson[12] noted that nicotine elicited short term stimulation followed by long term blockade. In order to obtain a valid estimate of nicotine actions in a whole animal, we sought to identify responses that would show stimulation and/or depression. The test battery that we have developed is described in detail elsewhere.[13] It includes measurement of: nicotine effects on respiration rate (an increase in rate is generally seen although some mouse strains show depressed rate before stimulation); locomotor activities as measured in a Y-maze (both the number of crosses into different arms of the maze and the number of rears onto the hind legs are measured, most mouse strains show depressed Y-maze activities), acoustic startle response (some mouse strains show enhanced startle response following nicotine, others are not affected or show modest depression), heart rate (nicotine elicits only a decrease in heart rate in the mouse) and body temperature (decreases in temperature are seen following nicotine). We have also measured sensitivity of various mouse strains to nicotine-induced seizures.

Recently, we have completed an analysis of nicotine sensitivity that used 19 inbred strains.[14] In these studies, we constructed dose-response curves for nicotine actions in each of the 19 inbred strains for all of the behavioral and physiological effects of nicotine that we routinely measure. In addition, we measured the sensitivity of the 19 inbred strains to nicotine-induced seizures following i.v. nicotine infusion.[15]

Figure 1 presents representative data for six of the inbred strains for the Y-maze crosses test. These six strains include three relatively closely related strains, the C57BL/10, C57BR and C58 strains, and three unrelated (to the C57/C58 family) strains, the AKR, CBA and DBA/1 strains. As should be evident from Figure 1, all of the mouse strains eventually exhibit a nicotine-induced decrease in Y-maze crossing activity, but the strains differ in sensitivity to this effect. ED_{50} values, the nicotine dose that decreased locomotor activity by 50%, were calculated for all 19 of the strains; these values ranged between 0.49 ± 0.21 mg/kg for the C57BL/10 strain to 1.89 ± 0 33 mg/kg for the BUB strain. Thus, mouse strains exhibit a 3-4 fold difference in sensitivity to the effects of nicotine on Y-maze crossing activity. ED_{50} values (mg/kg) for the strains depicted in Figure 1 are: 1.42 ± 0.31 (AKR), 1.07. ± 0.13 (C57BR). 1.43 ± 0.21 (CBA), 1.82 ± 0.08 (C58), 0.49 ± 0.21 (C57BL/10) and 0.93 ± 0.31 (DBA/1). Thus, the six strains presented in Figure 1 are representative of the 19 strains that we have examined.

The effects of nicotine injection on body temperature, measured 15 min. after i.p. injection, are presented in Figure 2. Nicotine elicited a dose dependent decrease in body temperature in all of the 19 strains. In this case, an ED_{-2} value, the nicotine dose that decreased body temperature by 2°C, was calculated from the dose-response curves for each strain. ED_{-2} values ranged between 0.55 ± 0.06 mg/kg for the A strain to 2.53 ± 0.08 mg/kg for the BUB strain in the 19 strains. Within the 19 strains, a five-fold variance in sensitivity to nicotine's hypothermia producing effects was seen. The ED_{-2} values (mg/kg) for the six strains presented in Figure 2 are: 1.37 ± 0.20 (AKR), 1.59 ± 0.32 (C57BR), 1.56 ± 0.36 (CBA), 2 07 ± 0.06 (C58), 0.61 ± 0.21 (C57BL/10) and 1.02 ± 0.26 (DBA/1).

FIGURE 1. Dose-response curves for the effects of nicotine on Y-maze crossing activity. Individual mice were injected with saline or one of several doses of nicotine and locomotor activity was measured for a 3 min period, starting 5 min after i.p. injection, in a Y-maze. Movement from one section to another was recorded. Each point represents the mean ± standard error of 6-12 animals.

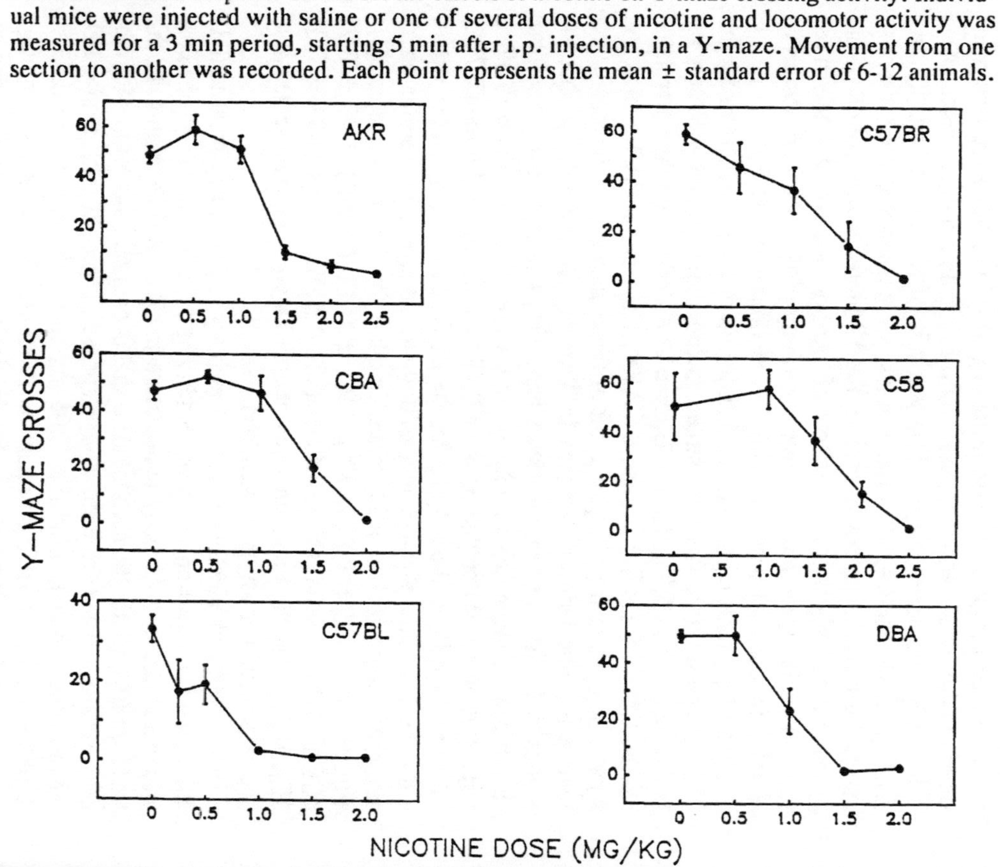

FIGURE 2. Dose-response curves for the effects of nicotine on body temperature. Individual mice were injected with saline or nicotine and body temperature was measured 15 min later using a rectal probe. Each point represents the mean ± standard error of 6-12 animals.

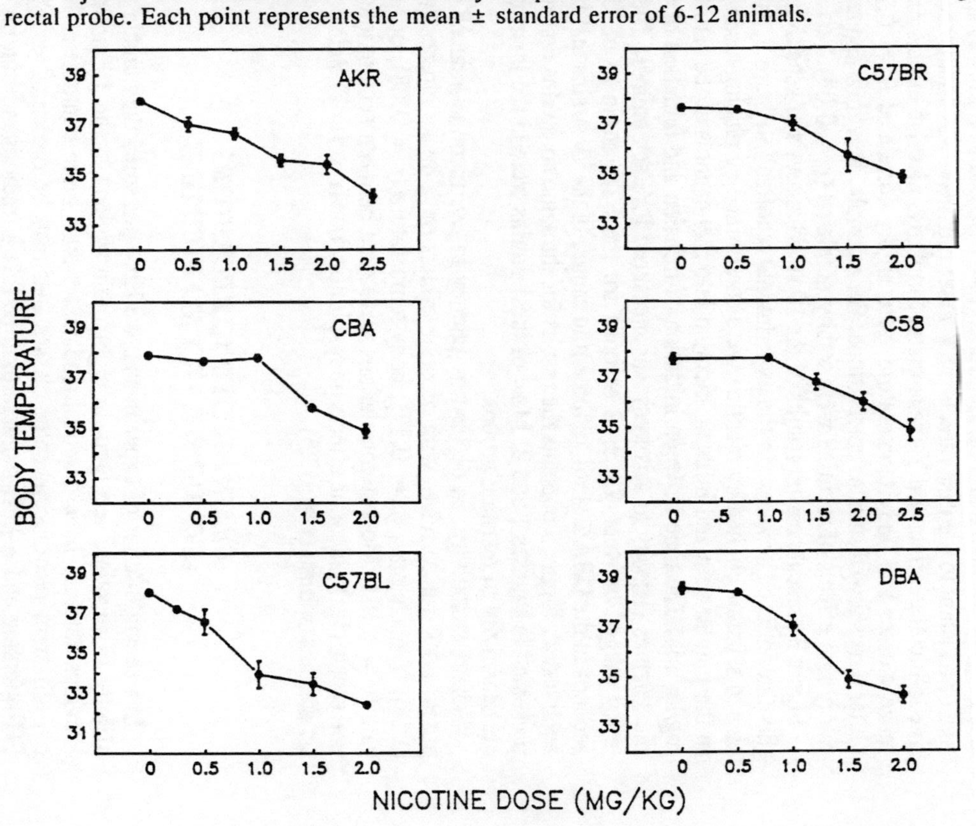

We have also measured the sensitivity of the 19 inbred mouse strains to nicotine's effects on Y-maze rearing activity, respiratory rate, acoustic startle response and heart rate. Subsequently, correlations between the responses were calculated. Nicotine effects on Y-maze crosses and rears were highly correlated among 19 strains (r = 0.93). If a strain was sensitive or resistant to nicotine effects on Y-maze crosses it was equally sensitive to nicotine effects on Y-maze rears. Similarly, nicotine effects on Y-maze crosses and body temperature were highly correlated (r = 0.72). Other tests showed smaller correlations. For example, heart rate and respiratory rate effects of nicotine were totally unrelated (r = 0.03).

Figure 3 presents partial results of the 19 strain analysis of sensitivity to nicotine-induced seizures. In the experiments reported in Figure 3, latencies to seizures elicited by nicotine were determined by placing a cannula in the jugular vein and infusing nicotine into this cannula at the rate of 2 mg/kg/min. The time between initiation of infusion and initiation of clonic seizures (latency to seizures) was measured for each animal. The latency ranged between 23 ± 2 seconds for the ST/b strain to 68 ± 8 seconds in the DBA/2 strain (a three fold range) in the 19 strains that have been tested. Figure 3 presents the results for the same six strains that were presented in Figures 1 and 2. Most of these strains were in the intermediate sensitivity to resistant groups.

Seizure sensitivity, as defined by latency to i.v. nicotine-induced seizures, does not correlate with nicotine effects on Y-maze crosses (r = 0.14), Y-maze rears (r = 0.17), body temperature (r = 0.08), or heart rate (r = 0.01). Modest correlations were seen between seizure latency and sensitivity to nicotine effects on respiratory rate (r = 0.47) and acoustic startle response (r = 0.25).

BRAIN NICOTINIC RECEPTORS AND SENSITIVITY TO NICOTINE

In a separate series of experiments, we have measured the number and affinity of nicotinic receptors in eight brain regions in the 19 strains.[16] Previous studies[17] have demonstrated that mouse brain contains at least two different nicotinic receptor classes that may be discerned using L-[^{3}H]-nicotine and α-[^{125}I]-bungarotoxin (BTX) in radioligand binding assays. Molecular genetic strategies have identified a minimum of four different nicotinic receptors in brain but one receptor subtype that contains so-called alpha-4 and beta-2 subunits seems to dominate in brain.[18] This receptor is likely measured with [^{3}H]-nicotine binding. The dissociation constants (K_D values) did not differ among the eight brain regions or

FIGURE 3. Latency to nicotine-induced seizures. Mice were infused with nicotine, intravenously, at a rate of 2 mg/kg/min. Latency between initiation of infusion and the development of clonic seizures was recorded. Each bar represents the mean ± standard error of 6 animals.

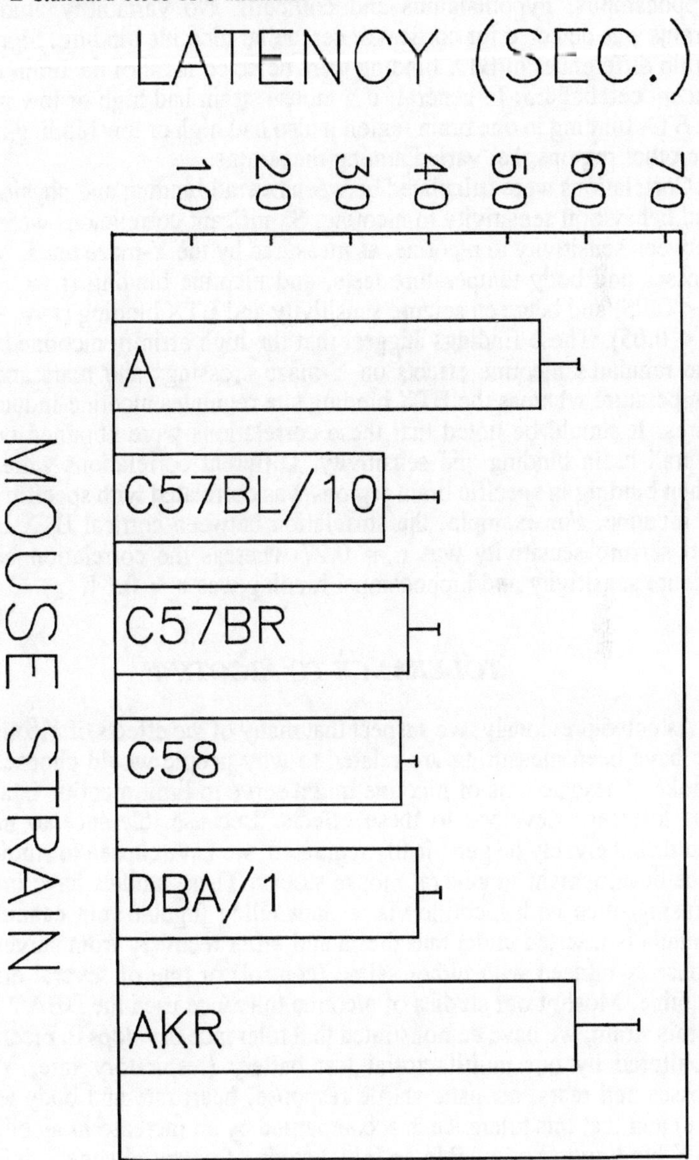

among the 19 strains for either nicotine or BTX binding. However, the 19 strains did differ in the number of receptors. Significant differences among the strains were found for nicotine binding in midbrain, hindbrain, hippocampus, hypothalamus and colliculli. No variability among the strains was detected for cortical or cerebellar nicotine binding. Significant strain differences in BTX binding were detected in all of the brain regions except cerebellum. In general, if a mouse strain had high or low nicotine or BTX binding in one brain region it also had high or low binding in all of the other regions that varied among the strains.

Correlations were calculated between overall binding and physiological and behavioral sensitivity to nicotine. Significant correlations were found between sensitivity to nicotine, as measured by the Y-maze rears, Y-maze crosses and body temperature tests, and nicotine binding ($r = -0.62$, $p < 0.05$) and between seizure sensitivity and BTX binding ($r = -0.63$, $p < 0.05$). These findings suggest that the high affinity nicotine binding site regulates nicotine effects on Y-maze crossings and rears and body temperature whereas the BTX binding site regulates nicotine-induced seizures. It should be noted that these correlations were obtained between overall brain binding and sensitivity. Different correlations were found when binding in specific brain regions was correlated with specific effects of nicotine. For example, the correlation between cortical BTX binding and seizure sensitivity was $r = 0.27$ whereas the correlation between seizure sensitivity and hippocampal binding was $r = 0.64$.

TOLERANCE TO NICOTINE

As noted previously, we suspect that many of the effects of nicotine that we have been measuring are related to why people would choose not to smoke. These actions of nicotine might serve to limit nicotine intake unless tolerance develops to these effects. Because tolerance to nicotine could conceivably be genetically regulated, we have chosen to study tolerance development in several mouse stocks. These studies have involved infusing mice with nicotine via an indwelling jugular vein cannula The cannula is inserted under anesthesia and, after recovery from surgery, the mouse is infused with either saline (control) or one of several doses of nicotine. Most of our studies of nicotine tolerance used the DBA/2 strain. In this strain, we have demonstrated that tolerance develops to nicotine, as monitored by our multifactorial test battery (respiratory rate, Y-maze crosses and rears, acoustic startle response, heart rate and body temperture) and that this tolerance is accompanied by an increase in nicotine and BTX binding in brain.[19,20] In an initial study of potential genetic influence on tolerance development, we compared the tolerance development of DBA/2 mice with C3H mice.[21] The C3H mice did not develop tolerance well; only at a 4 mg/kg/hr continuous infusion dose did we detect significant tolerance development whereas DBA/2 mice developed tolerance at much lower infusion doses.

Figure 4 presents the effects of varying chronic nicotine infusion doses on nicotine sensitivity, as measured by the $ED_{.2}$ value, in five inbred mouse strains (A, BUB, C3H, C57BL/6, DBA/2) as well as the selectively bred (for ethanol sensitivity) LS and SS mouse lines. As should be evident from Figure 4, some of the mouse strains, such as the C57BL/6, LS, and DBA/2 develop tolerance quite readily. Other strains, such as the C3H and SS do not develop tolerance to nicotine quite so readily, but they do develop tolerance at higher infusion doses.

The lower right hand panel of Figure 4 presents the relationship between initial sensitivity to nicotine and the threshold infusion dose required to elicit a 0.2°C differences in the $ED_{.2}$ value. A significant correlation between these two measures was seen such that mouse strains that are most sensitive to first time challenge with nicotine are those mouse strains that develop tolerance most readily. Resistant strains develop tolerance only at the higher infusion doses.

NICOTINE TOLERANCE AND RECEPTOR CHANGES

In previous studies, we have reported that DBA/2 mice develop tolerance to nicotine that is infusion dose dependent[19,20,21] and that this tolerance is accompanied by a dose dependent increase in nicotine binding. This increase in binding is seen in virtually all of the brain regions studied. BTX binding also increases with nicotine dose in DBA/2 mice, but higher infusion doses are generally required to produce this effect and changes are generally seen only in cortex and hippocampus.

Figure 5 presents the effects of varying infusion doses of nicotine on cortical and hippocampal nicotine and BTX binding in the five inbred mouse strains. It should be obvious that chronic nicotine infusion resulted in a dose-dependent increase in cortical and hippocampal nicotine binding in all of the mouse strains. Note, however, that for nearly every mouse strain maximal changes in nicotine binding occurred with infusion doses of 2 mg/kg/hr or less. The two inbred strains that showed the greatest increase in nicotine binding, the C57BL/6 and DBA/2 strains, were among the strains that developed tolerance more readily. The C3H and BUB strains develop tolerance poorly and these strains showed more mod-

FIGURE 4. Effect of varying nicotine infusion doses on sensitivity to nicotine's hypothermia producing effects. Mice of the various strains were infused with saline or nicotine (0.5-6 mg/kg/hr) for 7-10 days. Two hours after chronic infusion was terminated, individual mice were challenged with a dose of nicotine and body temperature was measured 15 min later. Complete dose-response curves were developed for each chronic infusion dose in each strain. The $ED_{-2°}$ value, the nicotine dose that decreased body temperature by 2°C, was calculated for each treatment group. These $ED_{-2°}$ values (± standard error) are plotted against nicotine infusion dose. Data from an earlier study that used DBA/2 and C3H mice[21] are presented for comparison (0). The lower right hand panel presents the correlation between initial (control) $ED_{-2°}$ values and the maximal infusion dose that elicited a 0.2°C change in the $ED_{-2°}$ value (threshold rate). Those mouse strains that were most sensitive to nicotine developed measurable tolerance at lower infusion doses.

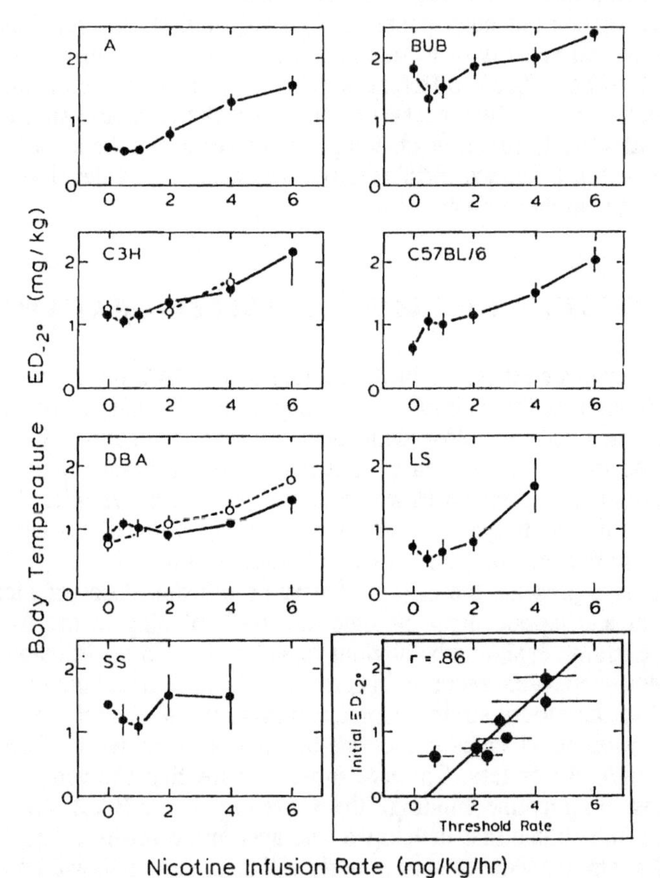

FIGURE 5. Effects of chronic nicotine infusion on L-[^{3}H]nicotine and α-[^{125}I]bungarotoxin (BTX) binding to cortex and hippocampus of five inbred mouse strains (C3H,○;C57BL/6,●; BUB,▲; A, Δ; DBA, □). Mice were infused with saline (0 mg/kg/hr) or 0.5-6.0 mg/kg/hr nicotine for 7-10 days . Two hours after infusion was stopped, the animals were injected with a challenge dose of nicotine and behavioral sensitivity to this dose was measured. Subsequently, the animals were sacrificed, the brains removed and dissected into eight regions and membrane preparations were prepared. Binding was determined in these membrane preparations using published procedures.[17] Each point represents the mean of 6-12 determinations. Binding changes represent alterations in receptor numbers; chronic nicotine infusion did not alter the K_D values in any mouse strain.

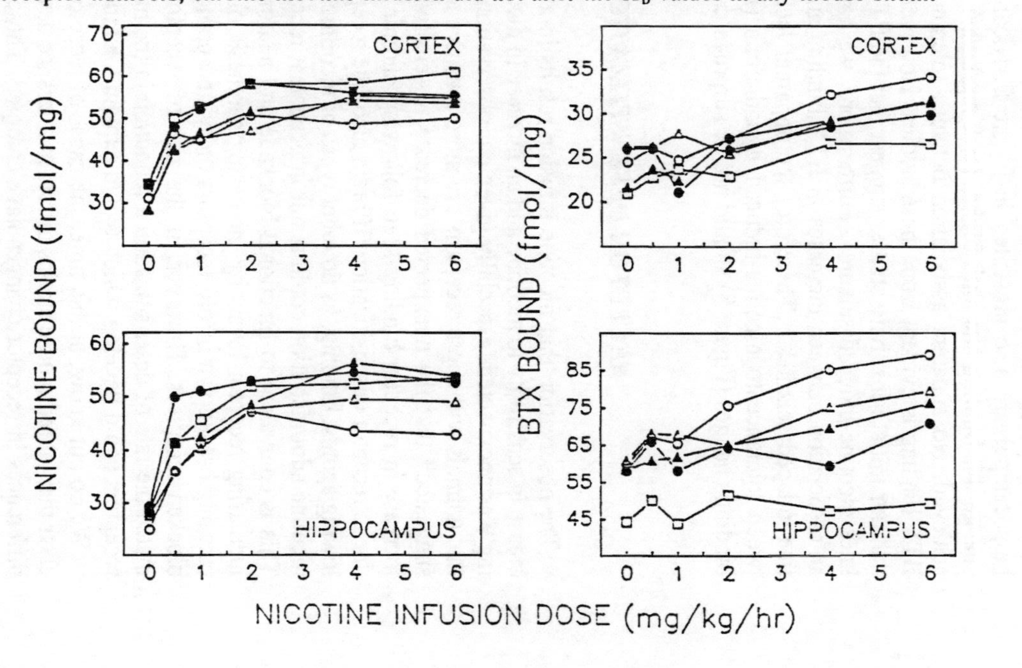

est changes in nicotine binding. Thus, it may be that a relationship between tolerance development and changes in nicotine binding exist.

The effects of chronic nicotine infusion on BTX binding in cortex and hippocampus are also presented in Figure 5. Nicotine infusion did not change this binding site until higher (> 2 mg/kg/hr) infusion doses were achieved. No apparent association between tolerance development and BTX binding is evident from these studies. However, it should be noted that our initial sensitivity studies suggest that the BTX binding site regulates nicotine-induced seizures. Furthermore, we have recently reported an association between increases in BTX binding and tolerance to nicotine-induced seizures.[22] Therefore, the apparent lack of association between tolerance to nicotine-induced hypothermia (Figure 4) and BTX binding changes (Figure 5) should not be surprising.

RECEPTOR DESENSITIZATION

The observation that nicotine infusion results in a dose dependent decrease in sensitivity to nicotine and an increase in nicotine and BTX binding was unexpected, especially given our observation in 19 inbred strains that animals with more receptors are more sensitive to nicotine. We have suggested[18] that the unexpected decrease in sensitivity coupled with an increase in receptor binding seen following chronic nicotine infusion is due to receptor desensitization. If brain nicotinic receptors desensitize following agonist binding, as do other types of nicotinic receptors, continual nicotine administration could result in persistent receptor desensitization. This is equivalent to functional blockade and neurons could respond by increasing receptor levels by increasing synthesis of new receptors, decreasing breakdown of old receptors or by uncapping hidden or partially blocked receptors. However, if the rate of receptor increase does not match the rate of desensitization a reduction in the number of activatable receptors could develop which would explain tolerance.

We do not know, at this time, the cause of receptor increases, but it is clear that inbred mouse strains differ. in tolerance development and strain differences in receptor changes have emerged. These differences may be due to differences in those processes that regulate receptor number and function, e.g., rates of desensitization-resensitization, rates of receptor synthesis and metabolism, and receptor capping and uncapping. Hopefully, once we understand these processes better we can provide a better explanation for inbred strain differences in tolerance development.

NICOTINE SELF-SELECTION

Very recently, we have initiated studies that may be related to the issue of why people might differ in beneficial or positive effects of nicotine. Preliminary results will be reported here. Figure 6 presents the results of an experiment where two inbred mouse strains, the C57BL/6 and A strains, were tested for nicotine self-selection. In these studies, mice were housed individually and were provided with two liquid-containing graduated cylinders (water and water-nicotine or 0.2% saccharin and saccharin-nicotine). The daily consumption of each of these fluids was recorded each day and the graduated cylinders were systematically switched so that place preference did not markedly affect the solution consumed. Every fourth day the concentration of the nicotine was changed.

As should be evident from the left hand panels of Figure 6, the C57BL/6 mice drank much more from the nicotine-containing solutions than did the A mice. This difference in consumption was seen in both the water-nicotine and saccharin-nicotine conditions. If, as seems likely, the saccharin is masking most or all of the nicotine taste, these results suggest, but most definitely do not prove, that the C57BL/6 and A mice differ in some factor that may be related to the rewarding effects of nicotine.

The right hand panels of Figure 6 demonstrate the C57BL/6 and A strains were identical with regard to total fluid intake for the water experiment. This was not true for the saccharin experiment. Saccharin administration increased total fluid consumption in C57BL/6 but not A mice. Nicotine addition did not appreciably change total fluid intake. However, nicotine addition did decrease the preference ratio (volume of nicotine solution consumed divided by total fluid consumption), but C57BL/6 mice showed a more gradual reduction in preference ratio than did the A mice.

CONCLUSIONS

Our results have demonstrated that inbred mouse strains differ in sensitivity to a first dose of nicotine that may be partially explained by differences in the number of brain nicotinic receptors. Mouse strains also differ in tolerance development following chronic nicotine infusion. The tolerance is accompanied by increases in brain nicotine and BTX binding. Subtle strain differences in receptor changes have been observed which may partially explain tolerance differences. The fact that initial sensitivity differences and tolerance differences have been observed in mouse strains suggests that humans may also differ in these factors. If sensitivity to

FIGURE 6. Self-selection of nicotine-containing solutions by C57BL/6 and A mice. Individual mice were offered a choice of either water and water-nicotine or 0.2% saccharin and saccharin-nicotine. Fluid consumption and body weight was measured for 4 days at which point the concentration of nicotine was increased; nicotine concentration ranged between 0 and 200 μg/ml. The left hand panel presents the average daily nicotine dose consumed for each of the treatment groups. The upper right hand panel presents the effects of varying concentration of nicotine on total fluid consumption; nicotine did not affect total fluid intake. The bottom right hand panel presents the effects of altered nicotine concentration on the preference ratio (volume of nicotine-containing solution consumed divided by total fluid intake). C57BL/6 mice clearly demonstrate greater nicotine intake than do A mice. Each point represents the mean of six animals for each 4-day block.

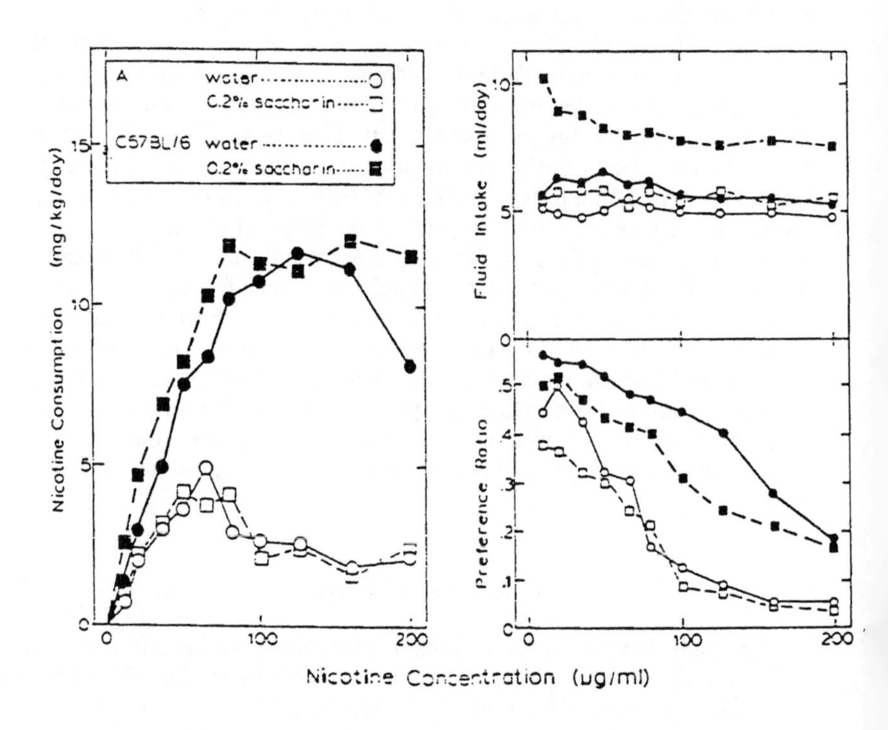

noxious effects limits smoking, it may be that initial sensitivity differences or differences in capacity or rate of developing tolerance contribute to those genetic factors that regulate tobacco use by humans. Lastly, our self-selection studies, if these relate to rewarding effects of nicotine, may indicate that genetic factors influence the rewarding effects of nicotine in humans.

REFERENCES

1. Fisher, R.A. Lung cancer and cigarettes. Nature. 1958; 182: 108.

2. Fisher, R.A. Cancer and smoking. Nature. 1958; 182: 596.

3. Friberg L., Kaij L., Dencker S.J., Jonsson E. Smoking habits of monozygotic and dizygotic twins. British Medical Journal. 1959; 1: 1090-1092.

4. Raaschou-Nielsen E. Smoking habits in twins. Danish Medical Bulletin. 1960; vol.7 3: 82-88.

5. Shields J. Monozygotic twins: Brought up apart and brought up together. Oxford University Press, London. 1962.

6. Conterio F., Chiarelli B. Study of the inheritance of some daily life habits. Heredity. 1962; 17: 347-359.

7. Pedersen N. Twin similarity for usage of common drugs. Twin Research 3: Epidemiological and Clinical Studies. Alan R. Liss, Inc. New York. 1981; pp. 53-59.

8. Stolerman I.P., Goldfarb T., Jarvik M.E Influencing cigarette smoking with nicotine antagonists. Psychopharmacologia (Berl.) 1973; 28: 247-259.

9. Pomerleau C.S., Pomerleau O.F., Majchrazak M.J. Mecamylamine pretreatment increases subsequent nicotine self-administration as indicated by changes in plasma nicotine level. Psychopharmacology. 1987; 91: 391-393.

10. Zacny J.P , Stitzer M.L. Cigarette brand-switching: Effects on smoking exposure and smoking behavior. The Journal of Pharmacology and Experimental Therapeutics. 1988; 246: 619-627.

11. Henningfield J.E. Behavioral pharmacology of cigarette smoking Advances in Behavioral Pharmacology, ed. by T. Thompson and P.B. Dews. Academic Press, New York. 1984; vol. 4 pp. 131-210.

12. Langley J.N , and Dickinson W.L. On the local paralysis of peripheral ganglia, and on the connexion of different classes of nerve fibers with them. Proc. R. Soc. London. [Biol.], 1889; 46: 423-431.

13. Marks M.J., Romm E., Bealer S.M., and Collins A.C. A test battery for measuring nicotine effects in mice. Pharmacology Biochemistry and Behavior. 1985; 23: 325-330.

14. Marks M.J., Stitzel J.A., and Collins A.C. Genetic influences on nicotine responses. Pharmacology Biochemistry and Behavior. 1989; 33, 667-678.

15. Miner L.L. and Collins A.C. Strain comparison of nicotine-induced seizure sensitivity and nicotinic receptors. Pharmacology Biochemistry and Behavior. 1989; 33, 469-475.

16. Marks M.J., Romm E., Campbell S.M. and Collins A.C. Variation of nicotinic binding sites among inbred strains. Pharmacology Biochemistry and Behavior. 1989; 33, 679-689.

17. Marks M.J and Collins A.C Characterization of nicotine binding in mouse brain and comparison with the binding of alpha-bungarotoxin and quinuclidinyl benzilate. Molecular Pharmacology. 1982; 22: 554-564.

18. Goldman D., Deneris E., Luyten W., Kochhar A., Patrick J. and Heinemann S. Members of a nicotinic acetylcholine gene family are expressed in different regions of the mammalian central nervous system. Cell. 1987; 48: 965-973.

19. Marks M.J., Burch J.B. and Collins A.C. Effects of chronic nicotine infusion on tolerance development and cholinergic receptors. Journal of Pharmacology and Experimental Therapeutics. 1983; 226: 806-816.

20. Marks M.J. and Collins A.C. Tolerance, cross-tolerance, and receptors after chronic nicotine or oxotremorine. Pharmacology Biochemistry and Behavior. 1985; 22: 283-291.

21. Marks M.J., Stitzel J.A. and Collins A.C. A dose-response analysis of nicotine tolerance and receptor changes in two inbred mouse strains. Journal of Pharmacology and Experimental Therapeutics. 1986; 239: 358-364.

22. Miner L.L. and Collins A.C. The effect of chronic nicotine treatment on nicotine-induced seizures. Psychopharmacology. 1988; 95: 52-55.

Is There a Common Biological Basis for Reinforcement from Alcohol and Other Drugs?

Frank R. George, PhD

SUMMARY. Vulnerability to substance abuse is an important emerging issue. A critical aspect of this phenomenon is the degree to which individuals who abuse one substance are likely to abuse other substances, alone or in combination with each other. The extent to which several distinct drugs will come to serve as positive reinforcers within genetically defined subjects defines their commonality. Questions in this area are directed at determining whether reinforcement from and abuse of alcohol and other drugs define variations within a single behavioral phenomenon, or whether reinforcement and abuse must be individually defined for each substance involved. Findings related to this commonality issue are now emerging from the areas of pharmacogenetics and operant drug self-administration. Previous studies have shown that ethanol can be readily established as a positive reinforcer in LEWIS rats, as well as C57BL/6J mice. In low ethanol preferring F344 rats, ethanol maintains significant but low levels of responding. Ethanol does not maintain lever pressing behavior in BALB/cJ mice, and is avoided in DBA/2J mice. Initial findings reported in this paper show that these genotypic patterns of

---

Frank R. George is affiliated with Behavioral and Biochemical Genetics, Preclinical Pharmacology Branch, NIDA Addiction Research Center, Baltimore, MD and the Department of Pharmacology and Toxicology, School of Pharmacy, University of Maryland, Baltimore.

Reprint requests may be addressed to Dr. Frank R. George, School of Pharmacy, University of Maryland, 20 N. Pine St., Baltimore, MD 21201 USA.

This research was supported in part by NIAAA New Investigator Research Award AA-06104/06924 (FRG), by NIAAA Grant AA-07754 (FRG), and by NIDA Grant DA-00944 (RAM). The author thanks Gregory I. Elmer, Richard A. Meisch, Mary C. Ritz and Tsutomu Suzuki for their outstanding technical and intellectual contributions to the research discussed in this paper.

reinforcement from ethanol appear to correlate highly with patterns of reinforcement from cocaine and opiates. From these findings it is concluded that (1) there exist important genetic determinants of drug reinforced behavior; and (2) drug seeking behaviors maintained by ethanol, cocaine and opiates may have at least some common biological determinants.

INTRODUCTION

Behavioral geneticists have at their disposal several conceptual and methodological tools which they can bring to bear on important issues related to substance abuse. These tools include the use of inbred, selectively bred and recombinant inbred rodent strains, in addition to experimental designs such as classical genetic (Mendelian) analysis and correlational studies. An important issue in substance abuse is the degree to which individuals who abuse one substance are likely to abuse other substances, alone or in combination with each other. The extent to which several distinct drugs will come to serve as positive reinforcers within genetically defined subjects defines their commonality. Behavioral genetic and pharmacogenetic methods are ideal tools with which to determine the commonality of drug-seeking behaviors across drugs within genetically defined individuals, as well as common biochemical substrates of these behaviors.

We now know that a number of drugs which humans abuse can serve as effective positive reinforcers across a range of non-human species including mice, rats and primates.[1-20] These findings indicate that drug-reinforced behavior, which over time can lead to drug abuse and dependence, has a strong biological basis. Recently, several reports have shown significant genetic influences on ethanol self-administration under operant conditions.[2,4,21-32] The results obtained in these studies indicate that genetic analyses are important in studies related to the understanding of drug reinforced behavior.

While there exist few reports on intake of drugs other than ethanol using genetically specified subjects, the existing data, almost all of which involves home-cage drinking of opioid solutions, do suggest that large population differences may exist with regard to drug seeking behavior.[5,33-43] Also, C57Bl/6J mice have shown consistently high preference and responding maintained by ethanol, opiates and most recently cocaine.[2,4,5,23-25,33,39,44-46] These findings provide foundation evidence that genetic factors play an important role in determining the persistence of non-alcohol drug taking behaviors, but to date there is only one published report of preliminary results showing genetic differences in operant self-administration of non-alcohol drugs.[5]

The integration of behavioral genetic and operant methodologies has great potential for increasing our understanding of the contributions and interactions of genetic and environmental factors in determining behavior. The methodology and principles of operant conditioning and pharmacogenetic analysis can be effectively combined to ascertain the relationship between one operant behavior, such as drug self-administration under fixed ratio schedules, with other operant behaviors, such as food-reinforced behavior, as well as with other, non-operant behaviors, such as locomotor activity. These comparisons can be used to determine the degree of common genetic control among these factors as well as to establish the extent to which one factor, such as neurosensitivity, covaries with another factor, such as self-administration. These and other issues, especially commonality of self-administration behavior across drugs, can be most effectively addressed by using genetically defined animals within self-administration paradigms.

The purpose of the present paper is to report initial results which demonstrate differences between several genetically distinct rodent stocks in drug seeking behavior, as well as within-strain commonalities in this form of behavior across three classes of highly abused substances, namely ethanol, cocaine, and opioids. Four genetically distinct rodent strains were used in these experiments, the LEWIS (LEW) and Fischer 344 (F344) inbred rat strains, and the C57BL/6J (C57) and DBA/2J (DBA) inbred mouse strains.

MATERIALS AND METHODS

Animals

Adult (10-14 weeks at start of testing) LEW (LEW/CRLBR), and F344 (CDF(F-344)CRLBR) male rats (Charles River) and C57BL/6J and DBA/2J male mice (Jackson Laboratories) were used. All animals were experimentally naive, housed individually in a temperature controlled room (26° C) with a 12-hr light-dark cycle (0700-1900 lights on), and given free access to Purina laboratory chow and tap water prior to initiation of the experiments. All animals used in this study were maintained in facilities fully accredited by the American Association for the Accreditation of Laboratory Animal Care (AAALAC) and studies were conducted in accordance with the Guide for Care and Use of Laboratory Animals provided by the NIH.

Operant Self-Administration Studies

Apparatus

A detailed description of the apparatus and procedures for the operant self-administration studies has been provided elsewhere.[2,5,9-11,28,32,37] In this system a spout is used to deliver a minute amount of liquid in response to a lick. An electronic circuit senses the small current (resistance adjusted to 5.0 megohms) traveling from the brass spout, through the animal's body to the grounded cage floor. As the tongue contacts the spout tip, a solenoid valve is opened momentarily to deliver a droplet of liquid (2.0 ul/lick for mice, 5.0 ul/lick for rats) directly onto the tongue.

Procedure

The procedures used to initiate lever pressing and drinking have been fully described elsewhere.[2,9-11,26,28,32,37] Session durations were 30 min. for mice and 1 hour for rats. To induce drinking, water bottles were removed and animals were given their food prior to or during the experimental session. After this training period, all animals had free home cage access to water for the remainder of the experiment. The rats and mice were initially reduced to 75-80% of their free-feeding weights and each drug was gradually introduced to the animals postprandially.

To determine if ethanol, cocaine or ETZ had come to function as a reinforcer, lever pressing behavior maintained by each drug was tested in the absence of food-inducement, and the animals received all of their daily food allowance after the sessions. A drug solution was made available for several consecutive daily sessions, followed by several consecutive sessions with vehicle (water). Retest conditions for each drug and vehicle were also performed.

Home Cage Drinking Studies

Apparatus

The animal's plastic home cage served as the experimental chamber. Each cage was equipped with a stainless steel grid top. Standard 100 ml drinking bottles with sipper tubes were used. Two additional cages with bottles but no subjects were used to control for evaporation and spillage.

Procedure

For the rat studies with cocaine, a limited access home cage two-bottle choice design was used, as described previously.[5,36] Sessions were run 5 days a week between 900 and 1200 hrs. The volumes consumed were measured at the end of each session by weighing the bottles. We tested whether LEW and F344 rats would consume greater amounts of a cocaine solution relative to a water vehicle. We measured intake of 0.57 mg/ml (-) -cocaine base vs. water during one hour home cage preference testing.

For the mouse studies with ETZ, a 24 hour forced choice single-bottle paradigm was used, as described previously.[38] Sessions were run 7 days a week. The volumes consumed were measured once every 24 hours. We tested whether C57 and DBA mice would consume greater amounts of an ETZ solution relative to water. We measured intakes of 1.25, 2.5, 5.0, 10.0 and 20.0 ug/ml ETZ and compared intake of these solutions to that of a water vehicle under identical conditions. All animals were weighed daily, and were maintained at 100% of their free-feeding weights.

RESULTS

Using adjunctive training and initiation procedures, all animals for both the operant and home cage studies showed large amounts of drug intake during training and thus had been exposed to the CNS effects of the drugs used in these studies. As a result, subsequent low intakes in any of the animals during tests for reinforcement could not be solely attributed either to a lack of association between drug consumption and resultant effects nor to aversive taste factors.

After training, and in the absence of presession food, liquid intake of cocaine solutions was higher in LEW relative to F344 rats in both the home cage and operant chamber test groups, and exceeded intake of water only in LEW rats. Liquid intake at 5.0 mg/ml during the home cage study is shown for LEW and F344 rats in Figure 1. The results suggests that orally delivered cocaine was serving as a reinforcer for LEW rats but not for F344 rats. Observations of the LEW rats and analysis of cumulative recordings indicated that most of the cocaine solution intake occurred during the initial portion of the test session.

The same strategies used previously to establish oral intake of drugs were effective in establishing ETZ as a reinforcer, but only for the LEW rats. Responding for ETZ significantly exceeded responding for vehicle only in LEW rats. F344 rats tended to avoid the ETZ solutions during the non-induced portions of the study. Patterns of responding for ETZ in both

FIGURE 1. Liquid intake in ul/g body weight at 5.0 mg/ml cocaine for LEW and F344 male rats during one hour non-induced home cage drinking sessions. Values are averages across ten consecutive days at this concentration. Cocaine solution intake is significantly higher only for LEW rats.

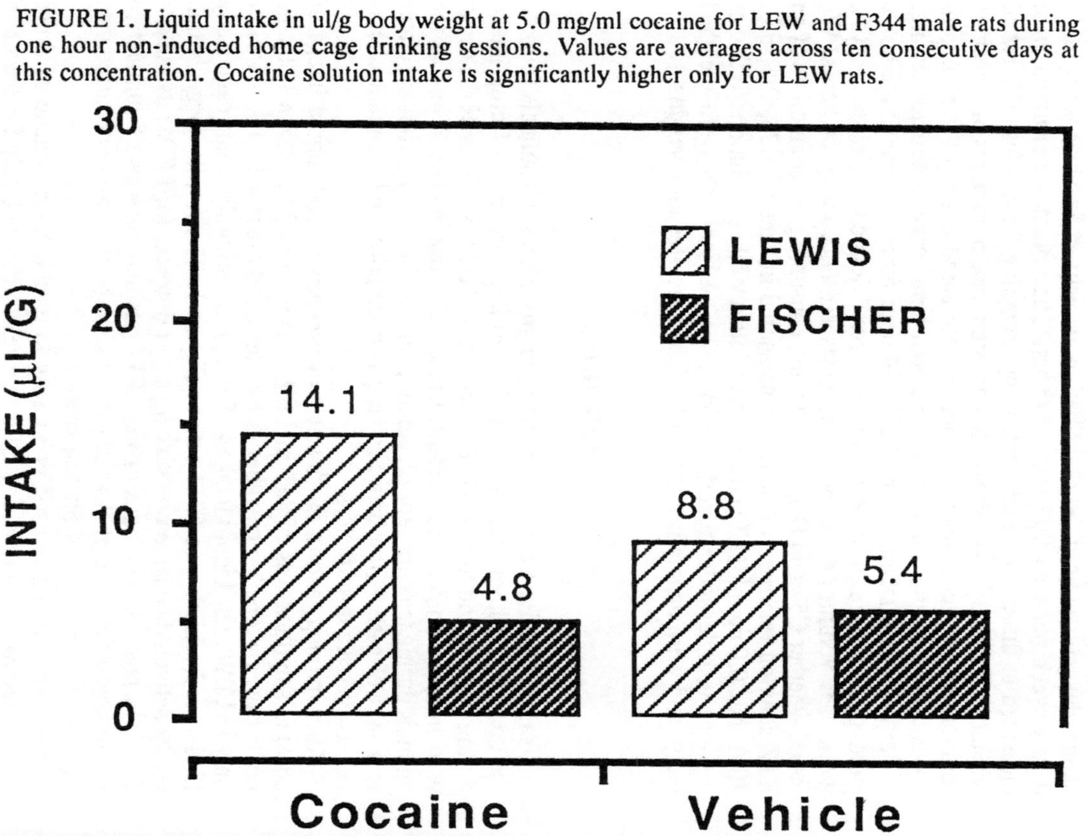

strains were similar to patterns seen with cocaine. Lever press responding by LEW rats was high during the initial portion of the test session, and decreased as the session progressed, i.e., was negatively accelerating, whereas responding by F344 rats was minimal and occurred sporadically over the course of the test session. Responding for 5.0 ug/ml ETZ vs. the water vehicle is shown for the LEW and F344 rats in Figure 2.

Liquid intake of ETZ solutions by C57 mice in the home cage forced choice study was consistently higher than intake of the water vehicle. ETZ intake was greatest at the 5.0 ug/ml ETZ concentration. Conversely, intake of ETZ solutions by DBA mice was very low, and was typically below the level of intake for water.[36]

Taken together, the results from these and other recent studies provide preliminary data concerning the degree of commonality of drug seeking behavior across multiple drugs and genotypes, as summarized in Table 1. Overall, the results suggest that a high degree of qualitative commonality exists across these genotypes and drugs. Genotypes which showed high intakes of ethanol also showed the greatest amounts of intake of and reinforcement from cocaine and ETZ. Conversely, genotypes which showed weak or no reinforcement from ethanol showed similarly low levels of intake of either cocaine or ETZ.

DISCUSSION

The demonstration of genetic differences in response to abused drugs is important for a number of reasons. First, the basic demonstration of genetic differences in responses to these substances illustrates the importance of genetic control in experimental research. This is a point frequently which has been all too often overlooked by investigators, journal editors and funding committees. The result has been a relative lack of incorporation of pharmacogenetic methods, despite their power, into other major areas of the pharmacological and behavioral sciences. This has also led to the propagation of misinformation concerning the role of genotype in experimental design and control. For example, a serious misconception regarding genetic control is the fact that many investigators routinely use Sprague Dawley rats because they believe this to be a strong level of genetic consistency and control, without realizing that animals with this particular stock designation are neither inbred nor outbred, and there is no definable genetic relationship among these animals.

Second, these findings provide a data base to be used for correlational studies with which we can examine mechanisms of drug action. A long term goal of the pharmacogenetics projects within our laboratory is the

FIGURE 2. Lever press responding during one hour test sessions at 5.0 ug/ml ETZ or water vehicle for LEW and F344 male rats. Values are mean number of responses across ten consecutive days at each concentration.

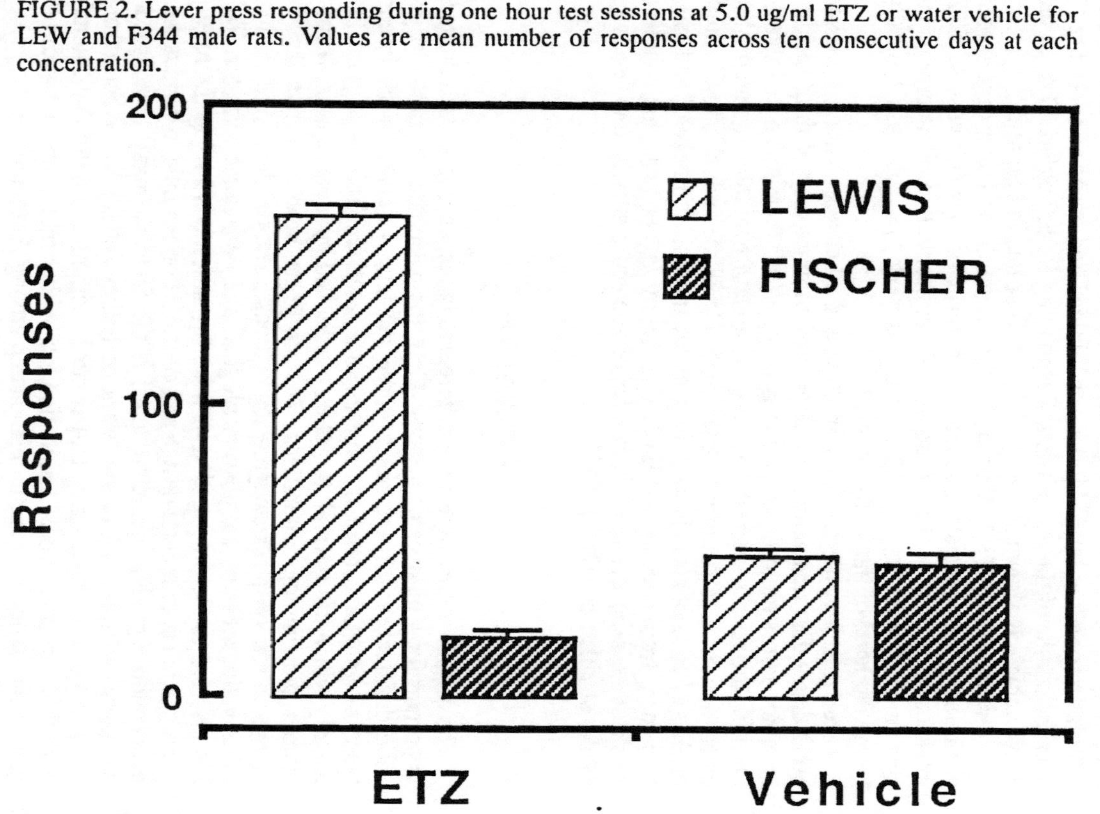

TABLE 1. Commonality of Self-Administration Behavior Across Drugs and Genotypes

Genotype	Alcohol	Opiates	Cocaine
Rats			
LEW	+++	+++	++
F344	+−	−−−	−
Mice			
C57BL/6J	+++	+++	+++
DBA/2J	−−−	−−−	NA

Note: Plus symbols indicate relative degree of positive reinforcement. Negative symbols indicate degree of non-reinforcement or avoidance. Three symbols is maximum response relative to all genotypes tested. NA = Data not available.

creation of a large data base matrix of rodent strains and drug effects. While this is an ambitious task, it will eventually be accomplished as more investigators begin to incorporate pharmacogenetic methods and controls into their research. The growth of a pharmacogenetic data base matrix illustrates a powerful advantage of this approach, namely that data obtained in one laboratory can be readily applied to findings from other laboratories, eliminating the need for endless repetition of basic findings. Thus, the use of genetic methods and controls is a very powerful approach to an efficient and economic buildup of a large drug-related data base.

A third point is that the demonstration of genetic differences in animal models of drug-seeking behavior suggests that there may exist human populations with differing degrees of biological risk for drug abuse. Realizing that individuals may differ in addiction risk, as well as understanding the biological factors related to risk can aid in the prevention and treatment of drug abuse. While it is unlikely that specific "addiction" genes exist, it may be that biological contributions to drug addiction result from interactions among several genes, each of which regulates a common and necessary biological system. In the case of persons at high risk for drug abuse, specific alleles would be present in a combination which is most conducive to making a drug an effective reinforcer.

These initial results from studies of drug self-administration across different drugs and genotypes are intriguing as they suggest that genotypic patterns of reinforcement from ethanol may correlate highly with patterns of reinforcement from cocaine and opiates. Thus, drug seeking behaviors maintained by ethanol, cocaine and opiates ma, have at least some common biological determinants. A detailed understanding of the commonalities of reinforcement across several genotypes and drugs would aid in our understanding of the complex problem of substance abuse.

REFERENCES

1. Carroll ME, Meisch RA. Oral phencyclidine (PCP) self-administration in rhesus monkeys: Effects of feeding conditions. J Pharmacol Exp Ther. 1980; 214:339-346.

2. Elmer GI, Meisch RA, George FR. Oral ethanol reinforced behavior in inbred mice. Pharmacol Biochem Behav. 1986; 24:1417-1421.

3. Falk JL, Samson HH, Winger G. Behavioral maintenance of high concentrations of blood ethanol and physical dependence in the rat. Science. 1972; 177:811-813.

4. George FR. Genetic and environmental factors in ethanol self-administration. Pharmacol Biochem Behav. 1987; 27:379-384.

5. George FR, Goldberg SR. Genetic approaches to the analysis of addiction processes. Trends Pharmacological Sciences. 1989; 10:78-83.

6. Goldberg SR, Morse WH, Goldberg DM. Behavior maintained under a second-order schedule by intramuscular injection of morphine or cocaine in rhesus monkeys. J Pharmacol Exp Ther. 1976; 199:278-286.

7. Griffiths RR, Brady JV, Bradford LD. Predicting the abuse liability of drugs with animal drug self-administration procedures: Psychomotor stimulants and hallucinogens. In Thompson T, Dews PB, eds., *Advances in Behavioral Pharmacology*, vol. 2. New York: Academic Press, 1979:163-208.

8. Henningfield JE, Meisch RA. Ethanol drinking by rhesus monkeys with concurrent access to water. Pharmacol Biochem Behav, 1979; 10:777-782.

9. Meisch RA. Alcohol self-administration by experimental animals. In *Research Advances in Alcohol and Drug Problems*, Vol. 8, edited by Smart RG, Cappell HD, Glaser FB, Israel Y, Kalant H, Popham RE, Schmidt W, Sellers EM. New York: Plenum Press, 1984:23-45.

10. Meisch RA. Ethanol self-administration: Infrahuman studies. In Thompson T, Dews PB (Eds.) *Advances in Behavioral Pharmacology*, Vol 1. New York: Academic Press, 1977:35-84.

11. Meisch RA. Animal studies of alcohol intake. Br J Psych. 1982; 141:113-120.

12. Meisch RA, Kliner DJ, Henningfield JE. Pentobarbital drinking by rhesus monkeys: Establishment and maintenance of pentobarbital-reinforced behavior. J Pharmacol Experimental Ther. 1981; 217:114-120.

13. Meisch RA, Stark LJ. Establishment of etonitazene as a reinforcer for rats by use of schedule-induced drinking. Pharmacol Biochem Behav. 1977; 7:195-203.

14. Samson HH. Initiation of ethanol reinforcement using a sucrose-substitution procedure in food- and water sated rats. Alcoholism: Clin Exp Res. 1986; 10:436-442.

15. Samson HH, Falk JL. Alteration of fluid preference in ethanol dependent animals. J Pharmacol Exp Ther. 1974; 190:365-376.

16. Schuster CR, Thompson T. Self-administration of and behavioral dependence on drugs. Ann Rev Pharmacol. 1969; 9:483-502.

17. Spealman RD, Goldberg SR. Drug self-administration by laboratory animals: Control by schedules of reinforcement. Ann Rev Pharmacol Toxicol. 1978; 18:313-339.

18. Weeks JR. Experimental morphine addiction: Method for automatic intravenous injections in unrestrained rats. Science. 1962; 138:143-144.

19. Wood RW, Grubman J, Weiss B. Nitrous oxide self-administration by the squirrel monkey. J. Pharmacol Exp Ther. 1977; 202:491-499.

20. Yanagita T, Ishida K, Funamoto H. Voluntary inhalation of volatile anesthetics and organic solvents by monkeys. Jpn J Clin Pharmacol. 1970; 1:13-16.

21. Sinclair JD. Rats learning to work for alcohol. Nature 1974; 249:590-592.

22. Waller MB, McBride WJ, Gatto GJ, Lumeng L, Li T-K. Intragastric self-

infusion of ethanol by ethanol-preferring and -nonpreferring lines of rats. Science. 1984; 225:78-80.

23. Elmer GI, Meisch RA, George FR. Differential concentration-response curves for oral ethanol self-administration in C57BL/6J and BALB/cJ Mice. Alcohol. 1987; 4:63-68.

24. Elmer GI, Meisch RA, George FR. Mouse strain differences in operant self-administration of ethanol. Behav Genet. 1987; 17:439-451.

25. Elmer GI, Meisch RA, Goldberg SR, George FR. A fixed ratio analysis of oral ethanol reinforced behavior in inbred mouse strains. Psychopharmacol. 1988; 96:431-436.

26. Elmer GI, Meisch RA, Goldberg SR, George FR. Ethanol self-administration in Long Sleep and Short Sleep mice: Evidence for genetic independence of neurosensitivity and reinforcement. J Pharmacol Exp Ther. 1990; 254:1054-1062

27. George FR. the use of genetic tools in the study of substance abuse. Alcoholism: Clin Exp Res. 1988; 12:86-90.

28. Ritz MC, George FR, deFiebre C, Meisch RA. Genetic differences in the establishment of ethanol as a reinforcer. Pharmacol Biochem Behav. 1986; 24:1089-1094.

29. Ritz MC, George FR, Meisch RA. Ethanol self-administration in ALKO rats: I. Effects of selection and concentration. Alcohol. 1989; 6:227-233.

30. Ritz MC, George FR, Meisch RA. Ethanol self-administration in ALKO rats: II. Effects of selection and fixed ratio size. Alcohol. 1989; 6:235-239.

31. Samson HH, Tolliver GA, Lumeng L, Li-T-K. Initiation of alcohol reinforcement in the alcohol nonpreferring (NP) rat using behavioral techniques without food deprivation. Alcoholism: Clin Exp Res. 1988; 12:308.

32. Suzuki T, George FR, Meisch RA. Differential establishment and maintenance of oral ethanol reinforced behavior in Lewis and Fischer 344 inbred rat strains. J Pharm Exp Ther. 1988; 245:164-170.

33. Broadhurst PL. Drugs and the Inheritance of Behavior: A Survey of Comparative Pharmacogenetics. New York and London: Plenum, 1979. 206 pp.

34. Carroll ME, Pederson MC, Harrison RG. Food deprivation reveals strain differences in opiate intake of Sprague-Dawley and Wistar rats. Pharmacol Biochem Behav. 1986; 24:1095-1099.

35. Crabbe JC, Belknap JK. Pharmacogenetic tools in the study of drug tolerance and dependence. Subst Alc Actions/Misuse. 1980; 1:385-413.

36. George FR, Meisch RA. Oral narcotic intake as a reinforcer: Genotype × Environment interactions. Behav Genet. 1984; 14:603.

37. George FR, Elmer GI, Meisch RA, Goldberg SR. Oral self-administration of cocaine in C57BL/6J mice and the relationship between intake and behavioral effects. J Pharmacol Exp Ther. submitted.

38. George FR, Goldberg SR. Genetic factors in response to cocaine. In: *Mechanisms of Cocaine Abuse and Toxicity*. Clouet D, Asghar K, Brown R, Eds. National Institute on Drug Abuse Monograph, 1988; 88:239-249.

39. Horowitz GP, Whitney G, Smith JC, Stephan FK. Morphine ingestion: Genetic control in mice. Psychopharmacology (Berlin) 1977; 52:119-122.

40. Meade R, Amit Z, Pachter W, Corcoran ME. Differences in oral intake of morphine by two strains of rats. Res Commun Chem Pathol Pharmacol. 1973; 6:1105-1108.

41. Nichols JR, Hsiao S. Addiction liability of albino rats: Breeding for quantitative differences in morphine drinking. Science. 1967; 157:561-563.

42. Satinder KP. Oral intake of morphine in selectively bred rats. Pharmacol Biochem Behav. 1977; 4:43-49.

43. Suzuki T, Otani K, Koike Y, Misawa M. Genetic differences in preference for morphine and codeine in Lewis and Fischer 344 inbred rat strains. Jpn J Pharmacol. 1988; 47:425-431.

44. McClearn GE, Rodgers DA. Differences in alcohol preference among inbred strains of mice. Quart J Stud Alc. 1959; 20:691-695.

45. McClearn GE, Rodgers DA. Genetic factors in alcohol preference of laboratory mice. J Comp Phys Psych. 1961; 54:116-119.

46. Rodgers DA, McClearn GE. Mouse strain differences in preference for various concentrations of alcohol. Q J Stud Alc. 1962; 23:26-33.

Genetic Determinants of Susceptibility to the Rewarding and Other Behavioral Actions of Cocaine

Thomas W. Seale, PhD
John M. Carney, PhD

SUMMARY. The role of genotype as a determinant of biologically based inter-individual differences in vulnerability to substance abuse has received little systematic investigation except in the case of alcohol. This report describes the use of an animal model, the inbred mouse, to identify and to characterize variants with inherently altered susceptibilities to the rewarding and other behavioral actions of cocaine. Among a battery of nine inbred strains chosen solely for their genetic diversity, genetic polymorphisms commonly occurred which altered the potency and/or efficacy of cocaine to induce conditioned place preference, oral self-administration, motor activity activation, seizures and lethality. These changes in cocaine sensitiv-

Thomas W. Seale and John M. Carney are affiliated with the Department of Pediatrics, University of Oklahoma, Health Sciences Center, Oklahoma City, OK and the Department of Pharmacology, University of Kentucky, School of Medicine, Lexington, KY.

Reprint requests should be addressed to: Dr. Thomas Seale, Department of Pediatrics, Room 2B-300 CHO, University of Oklahoma Health Sciences Center, Oklahoma City, OK 73190.

The research and concepts presented here were developed with the support of grants from the National Institute on Drug Abuse (DA 04028), the International Life Science Institute and the Presbyterian Health Foundation and by a contract (271-87-8133) from the National Institute on Drug Abuse. The authors thank Kathy Abla, Melissa Coxen, Frank Holloway, Michael Parker, Cao Wu, Paul Toubas and Lance Logan for their important contributions to the data and ideas presented.

ity generally were of a behavior-specific and pharmacodynamic nature. One strain, DBA/2J, found to be markedly hyporesponsive to the rewarding action of cocaine, also was hyporesponsive to the rewarding effects of amphetamine, etonitazene, phencyclidine, caffeine and procaine. We speculate that this strain has an inherent generalized appetitive defect. The frequent occurrence and large magnitude of inherent phenotypic changes in cocaine responsiveness which we have identified among inbred mouse strains now permits an analytical genetic study of processes underlying cocaine-mediated reinforcement.

INTRODUCTION

Anecdotal evidence and a limited number of controlled studies suggest that considerable inter-individual heterogeneity exists in the subjective effects, dependency risk, time course of dependency development and severity of the toxic effects associated with the use of psychomotor stimulants in man.[1-3] The mechanistic bases for these variations in responsiveness are only suspected at present. In view of the difficulty in controlling the large number of variables which impact on the human drug response phenotype, identification of genetic factors which influence vulnerability to cocaine or amphetamine dependence in man is expected to be a complex process at best. To undertake a systematic and comprehensive study of the influence of genotype on vulnerability to stimulant dependence, we chose to initiate these studies in an animal model in which genotype, environment and drug experience could be rigorously controlled. This paper describes our approach to identifying and characterizing variants with inherently altered responsiveness to cocaine. We have divided this presentation into three parts for clarity: (1) an overview of some pertinent general pharmacological issues; (2) a brief description of the characteristics of our model system, the genetically inbred mouse; (3) a summary of our current research findings.

1. General Considerations Pertinent to the Behavioral Pharmacogenetics of Psychomotor Stimulants

Significant inter-individual heterogeneity in the effects of a pharmacological agent is often found to occur in man and animals. For a given dose of a compound, some individuals may exhibit reduced effects (hypo-responsiveness) compared to the majority of the population (normo-responsiveness). Other individuals may exhibit exaggerated effects beyond those which occur in most individuals (hyper-responsiveness). The distribution of individuals among these three classes of responsiveness may or may not approximate a normal distribution. The outliers at the extremes of the response continuum are of special interest from both a conceptual and a practical point of view. These outliers may provide new insights into innate and environmental mechanisms which impact on susceptibility to one or more effects of a particular compound. In the case of licit substances, the occurrence of such outlying populations defines the frequency of individuals who may not benefit from the desirable properties of a medication or who are at increased risk for deleterious effects such as overdosing or undesirable side effects at the usual therapeutic doses. For illicit compounds, such a distribution might reflect differences in relative dependence liability, risk of psychiatric consequences, specific toxic effects, etc.

For a given drug-induced effect, be it physiological or behavioral, the action of the compound is usually dosage dependent and has a characteristic maximal effect. Heterogeneity in pharmacological responsiveness among individuals can reflect changes in the dose response curve. Changes in *potency* of the agent will result in either greater or lesser doses of the compound being required to elicit the same final effect. Changes in the relative *efficacy* of the compound also can occur. In this latter situation the final magnitude of the induced effect is significantly greater or smaller regardless of dose. Efficacy and potency changes may occur together or independently. Finally, a third general type of alteration in response, the occurrence of a qualitatively distinct effect of the drug, may occur in some individuals.

The acute as well as the chronic effects of drug administration reflect the complex interaction of innate factors, pharmacological factors and environmental factors. Innate factors include pharmacokinetic alterations (such as intrinsically reduced/increased rates of drug catabolism), pharmacodynamic alterations (such as changes in number of receptors for a specific neurotransmitter in one brain region) and biologically determined set point or endogenous rate for a type of behavior (e.g., intrinsic mood state, high/low basal activity rate, etc.). Innate factors may be inherited. Alternatively, such factors may be intrinsic to the individual yet not genetically transmitted. Pharmacological factors include issues such as route of administration, specific attributes of particular compounds and their analogs (e.g., half-life, toxic or behaviorally active metabolites, etc.) and previous history of drug exposure. Environmental factors also may influence the response to a drug in many ways. These changes may include altering its rate of catabolism or its biodistribution, modifying the capacity of the organism to respond at the neurochemical level (e.g., neurotransmitter depletion) and restructuring the options for expression of a drug response in the case of behavioral effects. Both interactions with the inanimate milieu and social interactions may be significant. Thus, individual differences in responsiveness to a pharmacological agent, such as cocaine, are likely to arise from very complicated interactions between factors intrinsic to the individual, pharmacological factors and environmental factors.

Such complexity, coupled with reticence of individuals to admit illicit drug use, probably masks the role of genetic determinants as risk factors in dependence vulnerability and in the expression of toxicity following exposure to psychomotor stimulants and other controlled substances in man. Precedent for the possibility that inherited traits may alter the relative susceptibility of an individual to the rewarding effects of cocaine or other illicit substances is based on a substantial body of evidence that the reinforcing effects of ethanol are influenced by inherited factors.[4,5] Hereditary predisposition to a broad spectrum of disease entities associated with abnormal behavior and/or abnormal function of the central nervous system is now well recognized.[7] The fraction of individuals becoming dependent on cocaine among all those individuals who have experimented with this euphoriant may include individuals who are inherently biologically vulnerable to its rewarding effects.

The processes believed to intervene between the acute, drug-induced activation of the reward response and the subsequent development of dependence following chronic drug exposure are themselves complex. As indicated in Figure 1, acute hedonic responses are experienced in the milieu of other drug-induced behavioral and physiological effects. Opposing processes which serve to negatively regulate the net response to euphoria may be as significant as the rewarding actions of the drug.[8] Polymorphic genes existing in the population may influence any one or more than one of these response traits. An array of variants with altered susceptibility to the acute rewarding effects of cocaine, as well as to chronic responses should be anticipated. Each of these might possess a somewhat distinctive phenotype depending upon the monospecific or pleiotropic actions of the variant genes. This consideration and the large fraction of the mammalian genetic repertoire uniquely devoted to the development, maintenance and function of the nervous system (30-40% of the genome, an estimated 30,000 to 40,000 genes in man)[6] make intuitively unlikely the existence of *only* one, single specific genotypic change which uniquely confers sensitivity or resistance to the acute hedonic actions of cocaine or dependence

FIGURE 1. Overview of the complex interactions which may take place from the onset of drug-induced reward to the establishment of drug-seeking behavior and dependence.

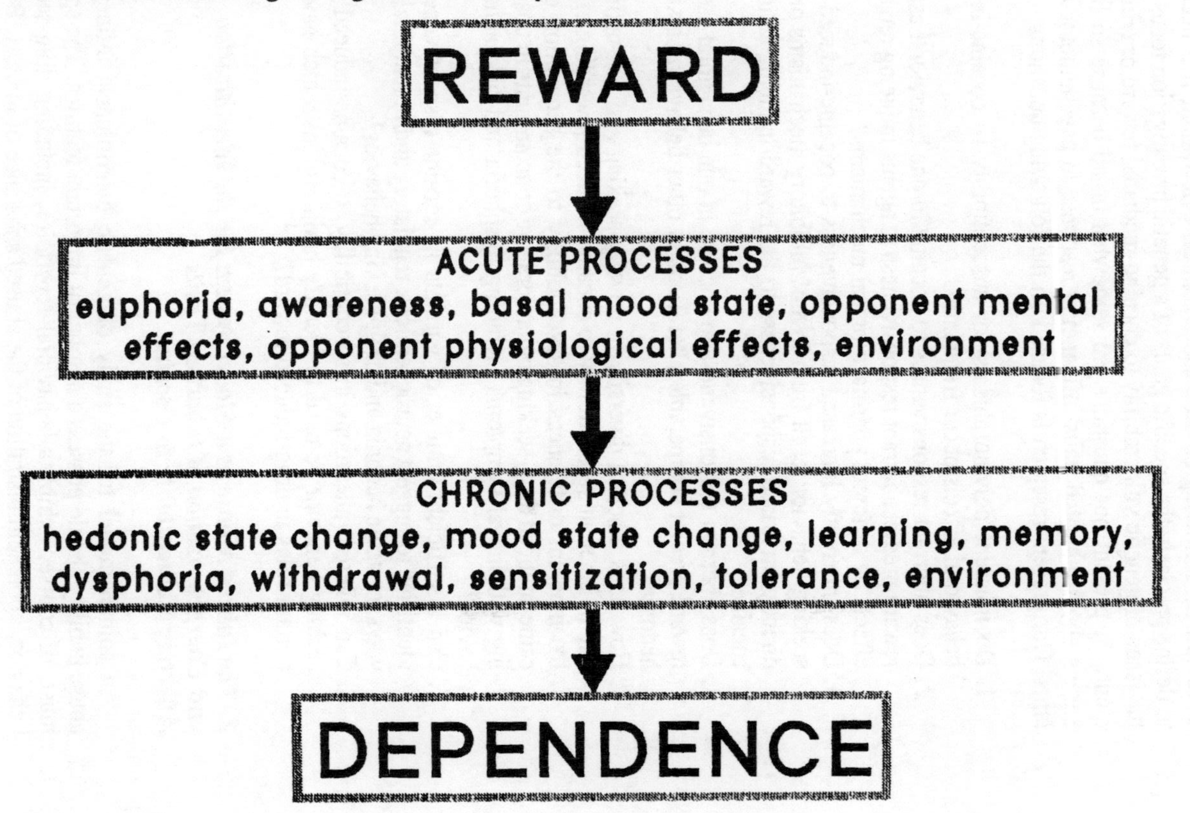

development following chronic use. From this viewpoint, it is necessary to define precisely the specific goals of a genetic investigation focusing on the issue of genetic vulnerability to cocaine-mediated reward or reinforcement. At present our questions are somewhat broad because so little is known about inherited traits influencing response to psychomotor stimulants. Our present research is focused on the following questions:

1. Do inherent polymorphisms for susceptibility to cocaine-induced behavioral effects occur frequently?
2. Does aberrant responsiveness to cocaine in one behavioral assay of reward predict aberrant responsiveness to agents inducing rewarding effects by different pharmacological mechanisms?
3. Does inherently increased responsiveness to cocaine-induced drug-seeking behavior result from loss of inhibitory mechanisms or from directly increased responsiveness to the reward-inducing actions of cocaine?
4. Does aberrant responsiveness to cocaine in one behavioral assay of reward predict comparable alterations in other behavioral assays of hedonia?
5. How does inherent diversity in novelty-seeking and risk-taking relate to inherent susceptibility to cocaine-induced rewarding effects?
6. Do inherent differences in susceptibility to the acquisition of cocaine-induced drug-seeking behavior have concomitants in post-dosing withdrawal symptoms including dysphoria and risk-taking behavior?
7. Can a sufficient number of variants in cocaine responsiveness be identified to suggest neurochemical, regulatory and/or temporal pathways for acute hedonia and drug-seeking behavior?
8. Can inherent alterations in susceptibility to cocaine-induced drug-seeking behavior be used to identify brain regions which have important roles in drug-induced reward?

2. The Inbred Mouse as a Model System for the Identification and Characterization of Inherited Traits Affecting Vulnerability to Cocaine

An animal model for the study of genetic determinants influencing abuse liability should possess a number of important features. The species must, of course, exhibit a behavioral repertoire, including drug-seeking behavior, upon administration of the abused substance of interest. Behavioral responses should be quantifiable and reproducible. The species must be mammalian, obtainable in large numbers with known genetic backgrounds and preferably commercially available. The choice of the species should be optimal for the discovery and maintenance of response variants. Strains either inherently hyper-responsive or hypo-responsive for drug-induced drug-seeking behavior should be reproducibly distinguishable from the response of typical normal (wild-type) mice. In addition, the model should possess features which facilitate genetic analysis. Inbred mice possess all of these attributes.

Inbred strains of mice are obtained by lineal breeding through brother-sister or parent-offspring matings. A strain is said to be inbred when such a breeding regimen is carried out for twenty or more generations. Inbreeding leads to homozygosis at virtually every gene locus. Therefore, inbred strains are usually considered to be genetically homozygous throughout their genome. Each animal within a strain is genetically equivalent to an identical twin. The genotype is preserved from one generation to the next. Death of an individual does not lead to loss of its unique genotype and phenotype. *Intrastrain* genotypic and phenotypic heterogeneity is low. The decrease in phenotypic variability within a strain results from the reduction in the contribution of genetic variance to the overall phenotypic variance. In contrast to the low intrastrain genotypic and phenotypic variation, *interstrain* genotypic and phenotypic variation is high. Inbred strains arising from different geographical and historical origins frequently have non-identical combinations of alleles at different gene loci. Therefore, although each inbred strain has the same overall genetic repertoire, several different allelic forms of a given gene and many different combinations of gene variants may exist between strains. Several hundred such mouse strains are commercially available. In addition, there exist technically sophisticated methods uniquely available in the mouse for the determination of the mode of transmission and chromosomal assignment of inherited traits.[9,10,11]

3. Identification and Characterization of Variant Strains with Altered Responsiveness to Cocaine

We have exploited the genetic diversity among inbred mouse strains as the source for variants with inherently altered vulnerabilities to cocaine. Certain genes are said to be polymorphic, that is, they exist in different allelic forms which occur at frequencies much higher than the occurrence of new mutations. If a gene is polymorphic in an outbred mouse population, then upon inbreeding different strains will, by chance, fix different alleles at a given gene locus. It is possible to determine how genetically similar or different two inbred mouse strains are to one another by comparing the identity of alleles at a number of polymorphic genetic loci. An example of such a comparison is shown in Table 1. The genotype of the C57BL/6J inbred mouse strain is compared to that of eight other strains in this table. Three hundred and twenty single gene loci for which polymorphisms exist in mice have been characterized in the C57BL/6J strain. The closely related derivative strain, C57BL/6ByJ, differs from its C57BL/6J strain of origin by only one gene out of the one hundred and three potentially polymorphic genes examined to date. In contrast, each of the other inbred strains differs greatly from the C57BL/6J comparator strain. Take the A/J strain for example. Ninety three of two hundred and forty eight genes have allelic forms which differ from C57BL/6J. If these genes are representative of all polymorphic genetic loci, then 37.5% of polymorphic genes differ between these two strains. Similarly, each of the other strains on average differs from the C57Bl/6J strain by about 40%. Regardless of which strain is used as the comparator, the strains are found to differ dramatically in their genotypes. This battery of strains was chosen to attempt to identify inherited variants in cocaine responsiveness because of their genetic diversity. There was no bias in strain choice based upon known basal or drug-induced behaviors. If inherited polymorphisms af-

Table 1. Genetic Relatedness Among Inbred Mouse Strains Based Upon The Comparison Of Polymorphic Single Gene Loci

Comparison Strain	Matching Percentage	Genes Matched	Genes Not Matched
C57BL/6J*	100	320	0
C57BL/6ByJ	99	103	1
A/J	62.5	155	93
AKR/J	58.3	151	108
BALB/cByJ	62.9	110	65
C3H/HeJ	65.7	163	85
CBA/J	59.5	150	102
DBA/2J	62.3	185	112
SWR/J	60.9	154	99

*Data are comparisons between the C57BL/6J strain and each of the other strains. Values are derived from data base of Dr. Thomas Roderick, the Jackson Laboratory, and include the data available as of 9/21/88.

fecting vulnerability to cocaine-induced reward occur in mice, then we expect a reasonable likelihood of detecting such variant responses among these different mouse strains because they differ so dramatically from one another across the spectrum of polymorphic gene loci.

In general our approach has been to identify a quantitative behavioral marker which is responsive to cocaine and to characterize the dose dependency of the effect of a comparator strain (for example C57BL/6J). Once this dose response curve has been shown to be reproducible, screening to identify variants among the other inbred strains of mice is carried out. Inherently hypo-responsive variants (compared to the C57BL/6J strain) can be identified by assessing the response of other strains to a dose of cocaine which elicits the maximal response in C57BL/6J mice. Hypersensitive variants can be identified by detecting strains which exhibit marked behavioral responses to doses which cause no changes or only threshold effects in C57BL/6J mice. This approach is efficient for the preliminary identification of variants with inherently altered drug responses. After demonstrating the reproducibility of the altered responses in the variant strain, pharmacological, neurochemical, behavioral and genetic characterizations can be carried out on other individuals of the same strain (which are, of course, genetically identical to the individuals used in the screening procedure and to each other).

A variety of markers for cocaine-induced effects *in vivo* are potentially applicable to our studies. These are summarized in Table 2. We have investigated many of these dosage-dependent actions of cocaine and have successfully identified variants with inherently altered responses for most of these actions. For example, large interstrain differences occur in the ability of cocaine to stimulate increases in locomotor activity. These differences include alterations in potency and efficacy of cocaine. Figure 2 illustrates the occurrence of a large decrease in efficacy of cocaine on this behavioral measure in the BALB/cByJ strain. The C57BL/6ByJ strain exhibits a characteristic 3-fold stimulation of motor activity following the acute administration of cocaine when vehicle-treated and cocaine-injected mice are compared. Maximal stimulation occurs at a dose of 32 mg/kg i.p. In contrast, the BALB/cByJ strain is markedly hyporesponsive. Its locomotor activity is not increased significantly above basal values at any dose of cocaine. This inherent alteration in vulnerability to the locomotor-stimulating effects of cocaine is of pharmacodynamic rather than pharmacokinetic origin. At cocaine doses which maximize the behavioral difference between the strains, the amount of cocaine present in the brains of the two strains is indistinguishable. This trait is inherited.

Table 2. Potential Markers For Cocaine-Induced Effects In Vivo

Behavioral Effects	
	Locomotor activity stimulation
	Stereotypy
	Place preference conditioning
	Oral self-administration
	Intravenous self-administration
	Intracranial self-administration
	Discriminative stimulus effects
Physiological Effects	
	Hyperthermia
	Hypertension
	Tachycardia
Toxic Effects	
	Hepatotoxicity
	Seizures
	Lethality

In the following section, we will emphasize newly obtained data on a marker of cocaine-induced drug-seeking behavior, the conditioned place preference (CPP) behavioral assay. Variants in this behavioral response to cocaine have been identified. Their phenotypes suggest that certain of these may result from a genetically determined alteration in the fundamental reward/hedonic response.

CPP is a behavioral bioassay for drug seeking behavior which can be quantitated and readily manipulated.[12,13] This response is a learned association of specific environmental stimuli (cues) with the positively rewarding or aversive effects of a drug. This leads to the preferential seeking out or avoidance of a particular environment in which an animal has experienced the administration of a specific drug. A positive CPP response operationally defines the appetitive or rewarding effect of a substance. It is said to occur when an animal spends a statistically increased amount of time in an environment with which drug administration has been paired. A variety of abused substances including opiates and psychomotor stimulants have been shown to induce positive CPP in the rat.[12,13] Only a single report has described differences between the responses of two strains of rats.[14] This assay has not been used previously to systematically evaluate the occurrence of inherent variations in vulnerability to cocaine-induced drug seeking behavior.

Our CPP experiments were carried out in wooden chambers divided

FIGURE 2. Illustration of an inherent strain-specific difference in sensitivity to a cocaine-induced behavioral change. Two strains of mice (n = 10 for each dose), C57BL/6ByJ and BALB/cByJ, received the same cocaine dosing regimen. The C57BL/6ByJ exhibited acute motor activity stimulation typically induced by cocaine whereas the BALB/cByJ strain was markedly hyporesponsive under the same conditions. Values were calculated by comparing activity levels over a 60 minute time interval post dosing in vehicle (saline)-treated and cocaine-treated groups.

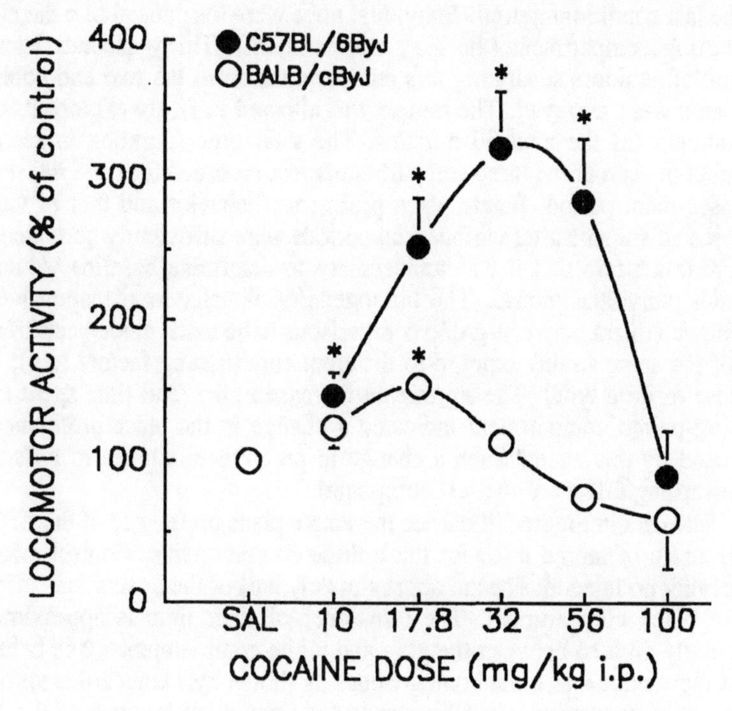

into three compartments which differed from one another in the presence of specific olfactory, visual and tactile cues. The center start compartment was gray with a solid wood floor and was separated from the end compartments by guillotine doors. One end compartment had a floor consisting of pine bedding and was painted white. The other end compartment had a floor consisting of wire hardware cloth over cedar chips and the walls were painted black. This configuration of cues was similar to that used by Bardo et al.[15] Each experiment was divided into two phases – a conditioning phase and an evaluation phase. During the conditioning phase, experimentally naive mice (n = 10 per dose or treatment regimen) were injected intraperitoneally with vehicle and placed immediately into one of the two end compartments for 30 minutes. At the end of the first 30 minute conditioning period, the mice were returned briefly to their home cage. Then they were injected with a vehicle or drug, as appropriate, and immediately placed in the alternate conditioning compartment for 30 minutes. Mice were not exposed to the gray (novel) chamber.

The evaluation portion of the experiment was conducted 24 hours after the last conditioning trial. Individual mice were introduced into the closed starting compartment (the gray compartment). Thirty seconds later the guillotine doors separating this compartment from the two end compartments were removed. The mouse was allowed to freely explore its environment for the next 30 minutes. The total time (duration in seconds) spent in each of the three compartments was recorded for the 1800 second assessment period. Innate place preference behavior and that of vehicle injected animals after various trial periods were sufficiently homogeneous within a strain that it was unnecessary to determine baseline values for each individual mouse. The homogeneity of behavioral responsiveness allowed direct between-group comparisons to be made among sets of mice (of the same strain) exposed to different conditioning factors (e.g., drug dose or drug type). The significant increase in the total time spent in the drug-paired compartment indicated a change in the place preference induced by this agent. Such a change in preference is taken to reflect the rewarding effects of the test compound.

The data in Figure 3 illustrate the innate place preference of the C57BL/6J strain of inbred mice for these three compartments. Control mice receiving no injections spend approximately half of the evaluation period in the black compartment. The remainder of their time is approximately equally divided between the gray and white compartments. The behavior of these mice was quite homogeneous as shown by a standard error of the mean of approximately 50 seconds for time spent in each of the three freely chosen compartments. Thus, with no injections of any kind, the mice do exhibit a marked preference for the set of environmental cues associated with the black compartment and are quite homogeneous in their distribution of time among the three compartments.

The rewarding effect of cocaine administration as judged by a positive increase in time spent in the cocaine-paired compartment of the CPP apparatus also is shown in Figure 3. Three separate experimental groups of mice are compared in the prototypic cocaine-responsive strain, C57BL/6J. Mice receiving three daily conditioning trials in which saline administration was paired with both the white and with the black compartment dis-

FIGURE 3. Comparison of place preference in C57BL/6J inbred mice under three conditioning situations. Control mice (n = 10) received no daily conditioning trials prior to their evaluation in the three compartment (identified as black, gray, white) shuttle box. Each compartment contained a different set of environmental cues as identified in the text. Saline-treated mice (n = 10) received injections of saline paired with placement in the black and the white compartments daily for three days. A third set of mice (n = 10) received saline injections paired with the black compartment and cocaine injections (1 mg/kg i.p.) paired with the white compartment. A statistically significant increase in mean time spent in the cocaine-paired compartment was observed when drug- and vehicle-treated mice were compared. Values are the mean ± SEM of the total time (in seconds) spent in each of the three compartments during the 1800 second evaluation period.

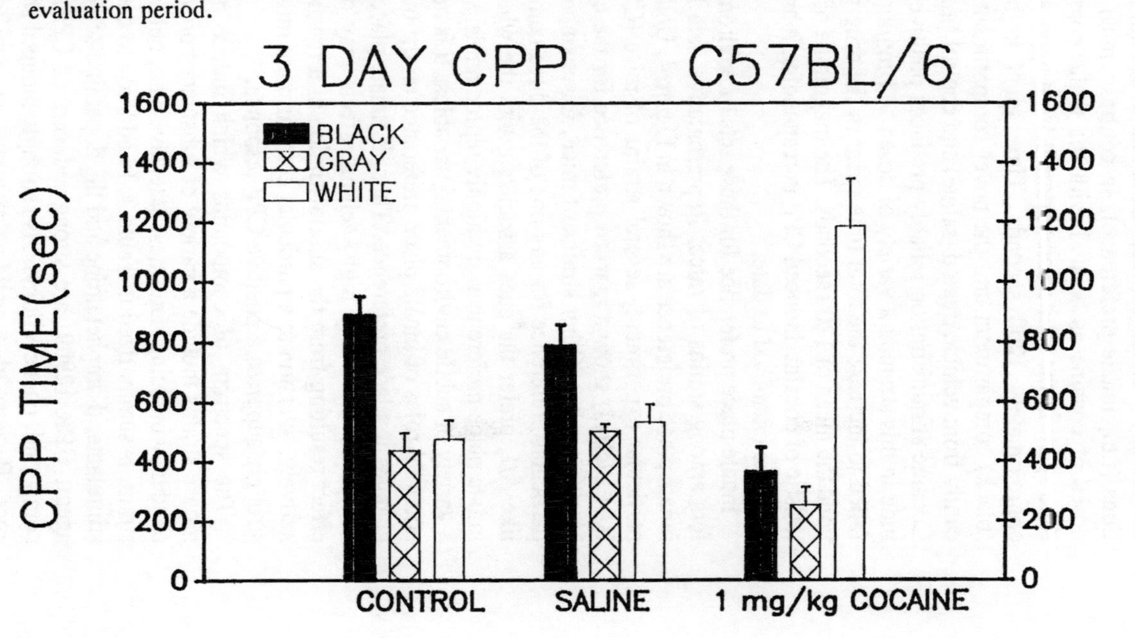

tributed their time on the subsequent test day in a manner which was statistically indistinguishable from that of control mice receiving no injections (i.e., innate preference). In contrast, mice receiving 1 mg/kg i.p. doses of cocaine associated with the white compartment increased the time spent in the white compartment from approximately 450 seconds to approximately 1200 seconds. Time spent in both the vehicle-paired (black) compartment and the novel compartment was decreased significantly from vehicle treated (saline) and control (innate) preference values. Cocaine administration reliably produces positive CPP of similar magnitude in this strain at a variety of doses > 1 mg/kg. Doses up to 32 mg/kg failed to increase the total time spent in the drug-paired compartment beyond the mean of 1200 seconds. The magnitude of this response is characteristic of cocaine-induced CPP in responding inbred mouse strains which we have examined to date.

Innate place preference for these sets of environmental cues clearly differs among strains of mice. Representative data for these differences in innate place preference are shown in Figure 4. Under the conditions of this particular experiment, several strains of mice (C57BL/6J, DBA/2J, and BALB/cByJ) show a marked preference for the cues associated with the black chamber. Other strains of mice, for example, C3H/HeJ, exhibit no particular preference for any one of the three compartments. Still others, like A/J, prefer the cues associated with the white compartment. These innate place preferences are highly reproducible when attention is paid to a variety of subtle environmental variables. It is necessary to consider the potential roles of innate place preference on the outcome of drug induced changes in place preference. Thus, if innate place preference for a given compartment is very high, ceiling effects may obscure a positive CPP effect resulting from the administration of a rewarding compound. Alternatively, aversion to a particular compartment might be so profound as to strongly suppress a positive CPP response.

The spectrum of compounds which induce positive CPP in inbred mouse strains include a variety of substances previously shown to be dependency inducing. Our most extensive data, obtained on the BALB/cByJ strain, is summarized in Table 3. In addition to cocaine, the psychomotor stimulants, d-amphetamine and the dopamine-selective reuptake blocking agent, GBR 12909, are strong inducers of CPP. The psychotomimetic compound, phencyclidine, also strongly induced conditioned place preference. Because phencyclidine may possess significant dopamine reuptake blockade properties, in addition to its non-competitive antagonist actions on the N-methyl-d-aspartate (NMDA) receptor, its actions on CPP may

FIGURE 4. Comparison of the innate place preference of eight strains of inbred mice (n = 10 each strain). The same sets of environmental cues (identified as black, gray, white) employed in Figure 5 were used in the three compartment shuttle box. Values are the mean ± SEM of the total time (in seconds) spent in each of the three compartments during the 1800 second evaluation period.

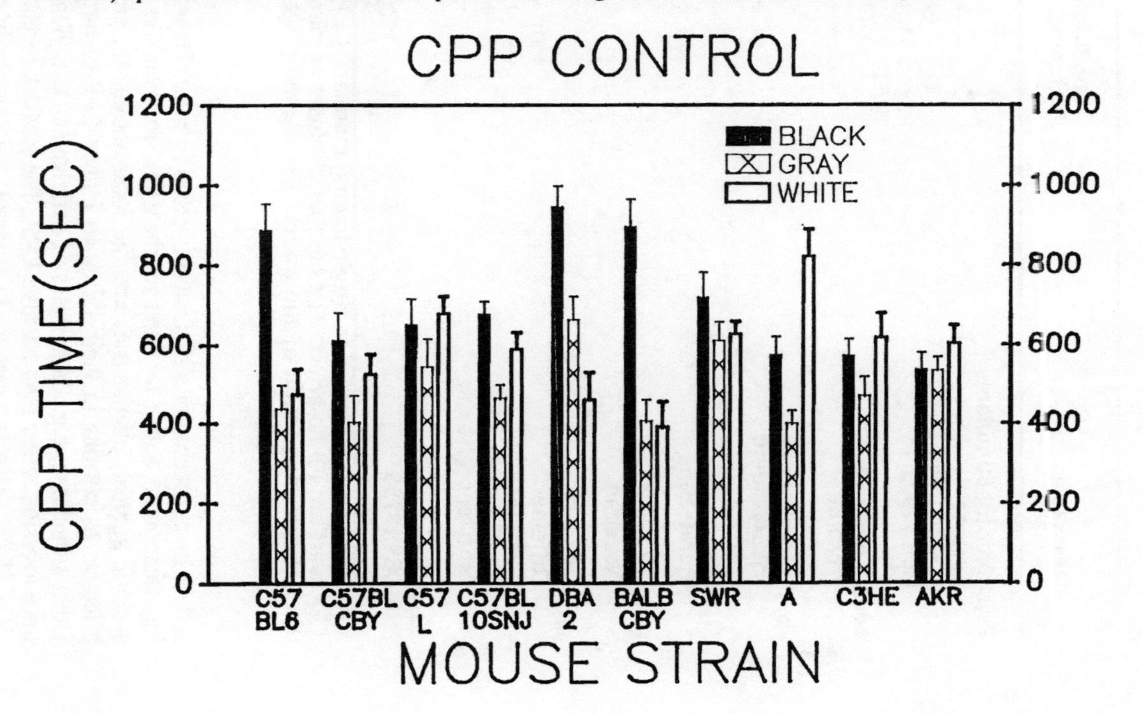

Table 3. Pharmacological Class Of Compounds Which Induce Conditioned Place Preference In BALB/cByJ Mice

Drug Class	Conditioned Place Preference Response
Psychomotor Stimulants	
Cocaine	+ + +
Amphetamine	+
GBR 12909	+ + +
Local Anesthetics	
Procaine	+ + +
Psychotomimetics	
Phencyclidine	+ + +
Opiates	
Etonitazene	+ + +
Benzodiazepines	
Diazepam	0
Other Stimulants	
Caffeine	+ or − − −
Theophylline	+
Paraxanthine	+
Pentylenetetrazole	−
Excitatory Amino Acids	
CGS 19755	− − −

CPP response is indicated in the following manner: (+) positive CPP; (−) aversion; (0) no effect. The number of pluses or minuses indicates the relative magnitude of the effect. Conditioning was carried out daily for up to 7 days.

reflect its psychomotor stimulant properties in mice. Dependency inducing compounds acting by other mechanisms, for example the mu-opiate specific agonist, etonitazene, and the local anesthetic, procaine, are as effective as cocaine in their ability to induce CPP of large magnitude. Other stimulants, e.g., high doses of caffeine and pentylenetetrazole, induce aversion rather than positive CPP. The NMDA receptor antagonist, CGS 19755, also is aversive. In contrast, the classically abused benzodiazepine, diazepam, fails to induce positive CPP under any of the dosing regimens which we have so far investigated (up to doses of 7 mg/kg i.p.).

The importance of these data is that the highly reproducible induction of positive CPP by a number of classes of abused substances allows the exploration of pharmacological mechanisms and the better definition of the phenotype in variants with altered vulnerability to cocaine-induced rewarding effects.

To date we have characterized the ability of cocaine to induce CPP in 9 strains of inbred mice. A high dose of cocaine (32 mg/kg i.p.) was chosen to attempt to identify variant strains which were hyporesponsive or aversive to the rewarding properties of this compound. The prototype cocaine-responsive strains, C57Bl/6J and BALB/cByJ, show large reproducible increases in time spent in the cocaine-paired compartment at this dose (an increase of 300 to 600 seconds, $p < 0.001$ compared to control animals injected with vehicle). This phenotype, Class 1, of strong positive CPP responders included two other strains of mice, A/J and SWR/J. The four remaining strains are dramatically different in their response to cocaine. One strain, C3H/HeJ, composing Class 2, showed a strong aversive response to cocaine. Four strains, DBA/2J, CBA/J, C57BL/6ByJ and AKR/J, compose phenotypic Class 3, hyporesponsive strains. These data identify the common occurrence of genetic polymorphisms for phenotypic vulnerability to cocaine-induced drug-seeking behavior among inbred mouse strains. These differences in cocaine vulnerability are inherent, highly reproducible and dosage dependent. For example, a dose of 32 mg/kg which induces a maximal CPP response in the C57BL/6J strain has no effect on the CPP behavior of the DBA/2J strain. Presently available data indicates that these differences arise from pharmacodynamic rather than pharmacokinetic changes. No differences have been found in the amount of cocaine present in the brains of strains which have differential behavioral responses to cocaine-induced drug-seeking behavior.

A detailed characterization of the behavioral and pharmacological phenotype of mouse strains with different inherent vulnerabilities to cocaine-induced drug-seeking behavior is underway. Table 4 indicates how informative such an analysis can be. Previously we indicated that the BALB/cByJ and C57BL/6J strains were the prototype cocaine responsive strains. While each of these responds readily and comparably to d-amphetamine and GBR 12909 administration in the CPP behavioral assay, and to etonitazene, the latter strain is markedly hyporesponsive to procaine-induced CPP. This difference is not pharmacokinetic in nature. It appears to be specific to the induction of drug-seeking behavior by local anesthetics. These data appear to separate the specific local anesthetic-induced mechanism for CPP from a more general response to cocaine.

Table 4. **Pharmacological Specificity Of Conditioned Place Preference Responses**

Compound	Inbred Mouse Strain		
	BALB/cByJ	C57BL/6J	DBA/2J
Cocaine	+ + +	+ + +	–
Amphetamine	+ +	+ +	– a
GBR 12909	+ + +	+ + +	–
Procaine	+ + +	–	–
Etonitazene	+ +	+ +	–

\+ Responsive – Hyporesponsive – a Aversive

They illustrate a specific inherent alteration in pharmacological responsiveness for the induction of drug-seeking behavior. In contrast, note the pharmacological non-specificity of the cocaine-hyporesponsive strain, DBA/2J. This strain not only is markedly hyporesponsive to cocaine-induced CPP, but is unresponsive to the opiate agonist, etonitazene, to the local anesthetic, procaine, to the dopamine-specific reuptake blocker, GBR 12909, and it shows aversion to amphetamine. These inherent differences to a variety of substances appear not to reflect some generalized pharmacokinetic abnormality in the DBA/2J strain. The pharmacological phenotype exhibited by the DBA/2J strain is consistent with a generalized abnormality in appetitive/hedonic responsiveness. Thus, marked hyporesponsiveness to cocaine can be associated with hyporesponsiveness to a variety of dependency-inducing compounds acting by pharmacologically dissimilar mechanisms. Two observations support the notion that the DBA/2J strain can sense the environmental cues and learn the association between drug administration and those cues. This strain does exhibit positive CPP following cocaine conditioning trials if a very high dosage is used (5 to 10 times that required for the induction of CPP in readily responding strains). Secondly, this strain shows rapid acquisition of negative CPP (aversion) following administration of aversive agents (e.g., a 32 mg/kg dose of caffeine). Its apparent pharmacological non-specificity in this behavioral assay does not arise from an incapacity to learn the behavioral task.

Another major issue is the behavioral specificity of the alteration in cocaine responsiveness. Representative findings on this question are qualitatively summarized in Table 5. Examination of this table identifies that each of five cocaine-mediated behavioral changes is highly polymorphic when the responses are compared among inbred mouse strains. These data also indicate that there is no necessary predictive relationship between hyporesponsiveness in one behavioral assay and the relative vulnerability of a strain to a second cocaine-induced effect. Among these five individual behaviors, each can apparently vary independently from the other. For example, the C57BL/6J and BALB/cByJ strains are highly responsive to cocaine-induced CPP. However, one of the two strains is strongly stimulated to drink cocaine-containing solutions while the other is not. Similarly one of these two strains is moderately stimulated in its locomotor activity by cocaine whereas the other strain is unaffected by similar doses. One is highly sensitive to cocaine induced clonic seizures whereas the other is hyporesponsive, yet both are equally hyporesponsive (as compared to other strains) to cocaine-induced lethality. For those strains which are hyporesponsive to cocaine-induced CPP (C57BL/6ByJ and DBA/2J), again, there is no relationship between cocaine-induced drinking, the effect of cocaine on elevating motor activity, and these strains are as hyporesponsive as the BALB/cByJ strain in sensitivity to seizure induction by this psychomotor stimulant. They have comparable susceptibilities to cocaine-induced lethality. Thus, genetic polymorphisms affecting several cocaine-induced behavioral changes occur in all combinations among mouse strains. The lack of correlation in relative responsiveness among these behavioral changes suggests that each trait is under separate genetic and/or mechanistic control.

CONCLUSIONS

The studies that we have described clearly establish that drug-seeking behavior, as defined by the conditioned place preference assay, is readily demonstrable in inbred mice following the administration of cocaine or other dependency-inducing substances. Variants displaying qualitatively and quantitatively altered responses for cocaine-induced CPP have been identified and occur commonly among inbred mouse strains. In general it appears that these polymorphic variants generally arise from pharmacodynamic rather than pharmacokinetic differences. Although we did not present the data here, the amount of cocaine and cocaine catabolites observed in the brains of mouse strains with non-identical behavioral responses did not differ statistically (whether unlabelled or ^{125}I- labelled cocaine was quantitated). Some CPP variants exhibit pharmacological specificity whereas others do not. Certain of the strains showing variant

Table 5. Comparison Of Susceptibility To Various Behavioral Actions of Cocaine in Four Strains of Inbred Mice

BEHAVIOR	INBRED MOUSE STRAIN			
	C57BL/6J	C57BL/6ByJ	BALB/cByJ	DBA/2J
Cocaine-induced CPP	strongly positive	hyporesponsive	strongly positive	hyporesponsive
Non-scheduled postprandial drinking of cocaine (POSA)	strongly stimulated	strongly stimulated	not stimulated	weakly stimulated
Cocaine-induced motor activity	moderately stimulated	strongly stimulated	no effect or inhibited	strongly stimulated, reduced potency
Cocaine-induced clonic seizures	highly sensitive	hyporesponsive	hyporesponsive	hyporesponsive
Cocaine-induced lethality	hyporesponsive	hyporesponsive	hyporesponsive	hyporesponsive

CPP responses are behaviorally specific in the sense that only a single measure related to the rewarding effect of cocaine is altered. Other strains with altered vulnerability to cocaine-induced CPP effects also exhibit similarly altered behaviors in other assays of appetitive behavior such as oral self-administration of cocaine- or amphetamine-containing solutions. There is no necessary relationship so far identified between inherent difference in intrinsic place preference or other innate behaviors and relative inherent vulnerability to cocaine-induced appetitive behaviors. Similarly there seems to be no systematic relationship between inherent alteration in vulnerability to appetitive effects of cocaine and other behavioral actions of this psychomotor stimulant. The existence of several different phenotypic classes of variants displaying altered vulnerabilities to cocaine suggests that different genotypic changes underlie each class. Formal genetic experiments are in progress to attempt to identify the number and chromosomal location of the genes which encode these cocaine-vulnerability traits.

REFERENCES

1. Nurnberger JI Jr, Gershon ES, Jimerson DC, Buchsbaum MS, Gold P, Brown G, Ebert M. Pharmacogenetics of d-amphetamine response in man. In: Gershon ES, Matthysse S, Breakerfield XO, Ciaranello RD, eds. Genetic research strategies for psychobiology and psychiatry. Pacific Grove: Boxwood Press, 1981:257-268.

2. Gawin FH, Kleber HD. Cocaine abuse in a treatment population: patterns and diagnostic distractions. In: Adams EH, Kozel NJ, eds. NIDA Res. Monogr. Ser. Vol. 61. Cocaine use in America. Washington, D.C.: US Governmental Printing Office, 1985:182-192.

3. Gawin FH, Ellinwood EH Jr. Cocaine and other stimulants: actions, abuse and treatment. N.Engl. J. Med. *318*:1173-1182, 1988.

4. Cloninger CR. Neurogenetic adaptive mechanisms in alcoholism. Science *236*:410-416, 1987.

5. Meisch RA and George FR. Influence of genetic factors on drug-reinforced behavior in animals. In: Pickens RW, Svikis DS, eds. NIDA Res. Monogr. Ser. Vol. 89. Biological vulnerability to drug abuse. Rockville, Maryland, U.S. Department of Health and Human Services, 1988:9-23.

6. Sutcliffe JG. mRNA in the mammalion central nervous system. Ann. Rev. Neurosci. *11*:157-198, 1988.

7. Baraitser M. The genetics of neurological disorders. New York: Oxford University Press, 1985.

8. Barrett JS. Behavioral approaches to individual differences in substance abuse. In: Galizio M and Maisto SA, eds. Determinants of substance abuse. New York: Plenum Press, 1985:125-175.

9. Bailey DW. Strategic uses of recombinant inbred and congenic strains in behavior genetic research. In: Gershon ES, Matthysse S, Breakefield XO, Ciaranello RD, eds. Genetic research strategies for psychobiology and psychiatry. Pacific Grove: Boxwood Press, 1981:189-198.

10. Taylor BA. Recombinant inbred strains: use in genetic mapping. In: Morse HC III, ed. Origins of inbred mice. New York: Academic Press, 1978:423-438.

11. Festing MFW. Inbred strains in biomedical research. New York: Oxford University Press, 1979.

12. Bozarth MA. Conditioned place preference: a parametric analysis using systemic heroin injections. In: Bozarth MA, ed. Methods of assessing the reinforcing properties of abused drugs. New York: Springer-Verlag, 1987:241-273.

13. Spyraki C. Drug reward studied by the use of place conditioning in rats. In: Lader M, ed. The psychopharmacology of addiction. New York: Oxford University Press, 1988:97-114.

14. Dymshitz J and Lieblich I. Opiate reinforcement and naloxone aversion, as revealed by place preference paradigm, in two strains of rats. Psychopharmacology *92*:473-477, 1987.

15. Bardo MT, Miller JS, Neisewander JL. Conditioned place preference with morphine: the effect of extinction training on the reinforcing CR. Pharmacol. Biochem. Behav. *21*:545-550, 1984.

Issues Surrounding the Assessment of the Genetic Determinants of Drugs as Reinforcing Stimuli

John M. Carney, PhD
Meng-Shan Cheng, MD
Cao Wu, MD
Thomas W. Seale, PhD

SUMMARY. A wide variety of drugs used in medicine and on a non-prescription basis have abuse liability. However, not all psychoactive drugs have demonstrable reinforcing properties either in animal models or in humans. In order to predict the abuse liability of a compound or to understand determinants of the abuse liability, several animal testing procedures have been developed. These procedures include tests for physical dependence, tolerance, disruption of ongoing behaviors, discriminative stimulus properties. and the direct or indirect assessment of the reinforcement. While tests for the production of tolerance and physical dependence may not predict abuse liability, they would significantly modify the abuse risk. This paper will focus on the methods available for the assessment of the

John M. Carney and Meng-Shan Cheng are affiliated with the Department of Pharmacology, College of Medicine, Chandler Medical Center, University of Kentucky, Lexington, KY 40536-0036. Cao Wu and Thomas W. Seale are affiliated with the Department of Pediatrics, University of Oklahoma Health Science Center, Oklahoma City, OK 73190.

Correspondence may be sent to: John M. Carney, Department of Pharmacology, College of Medicine, Chandler Medical Center, University of Kentucky, Lexington, KY 40536-0036.

The research and hypotheses presented in this manuscript were developed with support by a NIDA research grant DA-042108, and NIDA# 87-42108 research contract and by a grant from the International Life Sciences Institute/Nutrition Foundation.

The authors would like to thank Warren Landrum, Kathy Abla, and Raymond Hardwick for their contributions to the concepts presented in this manuscript.

reinforcing properties and the advantages of using genetically defined mice to better understand the determinants of the reinforcing properties and to isolate phenotypes that are hyper-responsive and hypo-responsive to the reinforcing properties of drugs under study. Examples of genetically determined differences are provided and areas of inadequate information are discussed.

Test designed to predict whether a drug will function as a reinforcer in humans rely on the observation that abuse drugs function as reinforcers in animal self-administration tests.[1] Exceptions to this generalization exist in both directions. For example, LSD-25 is not self-administered by experimental animals,[2] but is abused by humans.[3] On the other hand, procaine is reliably self-administered by experimental animals,[4] but does not have a significant abuse risk in man. The bases for these apparent inconsistencies need to be studied. In contrast to these exceptions, the vast majority of drugs found to be reinforcers in animal self-administration tests are also self-administered by human subjects.

Virtually all of the animal studies published on the reinforcing properties of psychoactive drugs have been conducted using outbred subjects. These studies are designed to be within-subject evaluations of a test drug, compared to vehicle controls. This design has been used extensively in self-administration studies and has been successful because is was recognized early on that there can be large interindividual differences in both the potency of a test compound (the effective dose range) and in the magnitude or amount of self-administration (maximal effect or efficacy) at a selected dose. In an effort to develop a systematic, predictive, approach to testing drugs that may have abuse liability, profiles of the characteristic properties of drugs of abuse have been discussed.[5-7] These drugs share many common behavioral effects, including: dose-related stimulation and depression of spontaneous locomotor activity, disruption of operant behavior, production of discriminative stimulus properties, production of physical dependence and/or tolerance. Other than the effect of maintaining self-administration behaviors, it is not well understood how (or whether) the other effects described are functionally linked to the determinants of the self-administration behaviors. One of the major difficulties is that each of the other effects also may be under complex genetic control, which increases the probability of a chance association of two or more traits. Thus, subjects that have the same drug responsiveness may in fact represent two or more populations of genetic backgrounds. This level of uncertainty makes the development of a successful strategy to characterize and isolate the reinforcement responsiveness phenotypes unlikely to succeed in randomly bred animals. The use of genetically defined mice offers an opportunity to reduce the intra-group variability. This paper will discuss some of the approaches employed in inbred mice to characterize the genetic determinants of drugs as reinforcers. It is not the purpose of this paper to provide an exhaustive review of the psychopharmacogenetic literature. Rather, the intent of this review is to discuss the methods of characterizing the reinforcing effects abused drugs and to demonstrate the advantages of using genetically defined mice in dissecting the component processes involved.

BEHAVIORAL EFFECTS OF DRUGS IN INBRED MICE

An extensive data base has been established for the effects of drugs on unconditioned behaviors. Inherent differences in responsiveness to opiates, sedatives, stimulants and ethanol have been described.[8-12] One of the dangers in generalizing these results is that the factors that determine responsiveness to drug "X" may not be responsible for determining responsiveness to drug "Y." This is often the case when then two drugs are in functionally different pharmacological classes. However, it also may be true when the compounds share the same presumed mechanism of action. A good example is the comparison of responsiveness to caffeine and theophylline. We have previously demonstrated that SWR/J mice are refractory to the behavioral stimulant effects of caffeine and theophylline.[13,14] The CBA/J mouse demonstrates dose-related increases in spontaneous locomotor activity. The presumed mechanism of action for this effect is blockade of brain adenosine receptors.[15] A logical assumption from the neurochemical data and the initial behavioral genetic data is that responsiveness to caffeine should predict responsiveness to theophylline. A corollary to this hypothesis is that responsiveness to the two methylxanthines is under identical genetic control. However, when responsiveness to the two xanthines was determined in the F2-generation cross of the these two strains, there was no significant correlation. These data indicate that some or all of the genetic determinants of responsiveness to theophylline are not identical to the factors that determine caffeine responsiveness.

If the genetic determinants of the reinforcing effects of drugs are to be isolated and their gene products characterized, then it is crucial that the pharmacological specificity and the efficacy be determined for those behavioral effects that co-segregrate and are to be used as screening tools prior to the direct assessment of the reinforcing stimulus properties. Unconditioned behaviors have been the primary screening tools for identifying genetic diversity in responsiveness to drugs. However, the literature on the operant behavioral effects of drugs provides numerous examples of how the schedule of reinforcement and the conditions of drug delivery can strongly influence the observed effects.[16] For example, under a fixed-interval schedule of food reward morphine, pentabarbital and amphetamine increase responding.[16,17] In contrast, responding under a fixed ratio schedule is decreased by these same drugs. Thus, the.same drug, in the same subject, in the same test session, at the same blood level of drug will produce qualitatively different behavioral effects. Schedule dependent differences in the effects of drugs have been demonstrated in human subjects, non-human primates. cats, pigeons, rats and mice. It is important to note that the rates and patterns of behavior under these schedules of reinforcement are essentially identical for all of the subjects studied. Studies in mice have demonstrated orderly effects of prototype psychoactive drugs on fixed-interval, fixed-ratio (FIFR) responding that are qualitatively similar to effects observed in man and laboratory animals.[18-21] However, comparison of different strains for qualitative or quantitative differences have not been reported. In particular, comparisons of responsiveness to the effects of drugs on unconditioned behavior to the effects of the same drugs on operant behaviors are lacking. For example, it is important to determine if the pattern of morphine responsiveness for locomotor activity predicts responsiveness to morphine under FIFR schedules of reinforcement. Using locomotor activity, C57BL/6J mice demonstrate a robust stimulation of activity, DBA/2J are decreased and A/J mice are unaffected.[9,22,23,24] Studies using operant behavior are considerably more labor intensive, but they are necessary if we are to carefully and systematically characterize the genetic determinants of responsiveness to the range of behavioral effects produced by drugs of abuse.

ASSESSMENT OF REINFORCING PROPERTIES

A number of different procedures have been developed to characterize the potential reinforcing properties of drugs. These procedures involve different levels of instrumental and classical conditioning. It should be pointed out that these different procedures do not necessarily measure the same things. Thus, the identification of a positive effect in one test procedure does not necessarily guarantee that the same compound will result in the identification of positive reinforcing effects in a different procedure. Of course, if a series of different procedures result in the same conclusion this increases the likelihood that the compound does function as a positive reinforcer and has a degree of abuse liability risk.

ORAL SELF-ADMINISTRATION PROCEDURES

There are basically three types of oral self-administration procedures. The first is oral self-administration using a single source of fluid to generate high levels of drug intake.[10,25] While this approach may result in a substantial amount of drug ingestion, there are a number of issues that complicate its interpretation. There may in fact be a reduction in the total fluid consumption as a result of the addition of the drug to the drinking water. The stress of reduced water intake may modify the effects of the drug and the pattern of drug intake. In addition, if the drug under study stimulates behavior, it may increase or decrease its own consumption. Other effects (such as diuresis. sedation. taste aversion) also will influence the extent of drug ingestion. An alternative approach is to use two drinking water sources, one with drug and one without drug. Often the drug is dissolved in a saccharin/water solution in order to insure that adequate experience with the drug solution occurs prior to progressive removal (fading) of the saccharin from the water. For example, when etonitazene (a potent narcotic) was added to a 0.2% saccharin/water solution both C57BL/6J mice and DBA/2J mice demonstrated a dose-related increase in consumption as the concentration was increased (Figure 1). However, the extent of the intake at the higher end of the concentration range was markedly different for the two strains. The markedly higher intake of etonitazene in the C57BL mice was quite stable and consistent. When saccharin was removed from the etonitazene solution, the intake remained high for the C57BL mice (Figure 2). Based upon these results there are two hypotheses that could account for such differences. First, the C57BL mice possess the responsive receptor systems that mediate the positive rewarding effects and the DBA are deficient in these systems. Second, the DBA mice possess the responsive systems that mediate the aversive effects (e.g., sedation, conditioned taste aversion, etc.) and the C57BL mice are less responsive. It is important to point out that the differences in intake of etonitazene parallels the responsiveness pattern for changes in locomotor activity in these two strains.

A second procedure to induce oral intake of drug solutions is schedule-induced polydypsia.[26-29] Under such a procedure a small amount of food (e.g., 45 mg food pellet) is delivered into a food hopper at regular intervals. Water or drug solution s are freely available during the experimental session. The periodic delivery of the food pellet elicits drinking. Falk and

FIGURE 1. Inherent differences in oral consumption of etonitazene in a 0.2% saccharin/water solution under a 2-bottle choice procedure. Drug solutions and water only were available in individual drinking bottles. The position of the bottle was switched daily in order to control for position preference. Total amount of drug ingested was determined for each day (23.5 hrs = 1 day). Each of the etonitazene concentrations was tested for 10 successive days at each concentration. Data are presented as the mean (± S.E.) of the last 3 days for 10-12 mice at each of the etonitazene concentrations. Etonitazene concentrations were tested in an ascending concentration series.

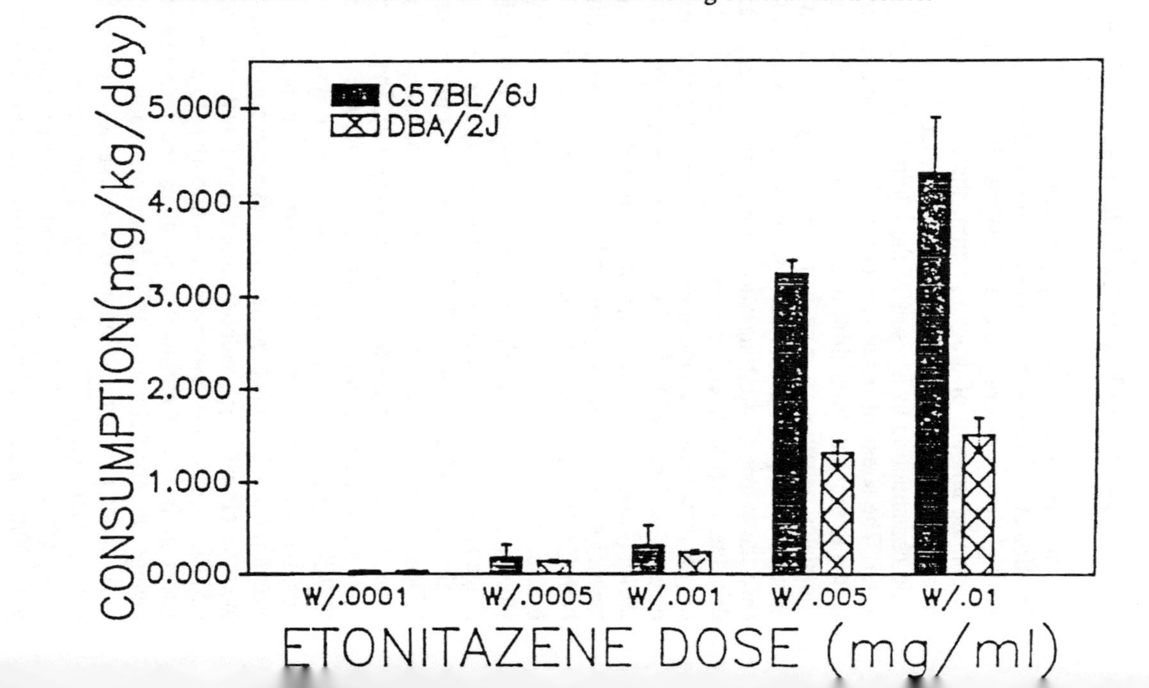

FIGURE 2. Strain related difference in oral etonitazene consumption across decreasing concentrations of saccharin and in water alone. Data are the mean ± S. E. of 10-12 mice on the last day (each saccharin concentration was studied for 3 consecutive days) at each saccharin concentration.

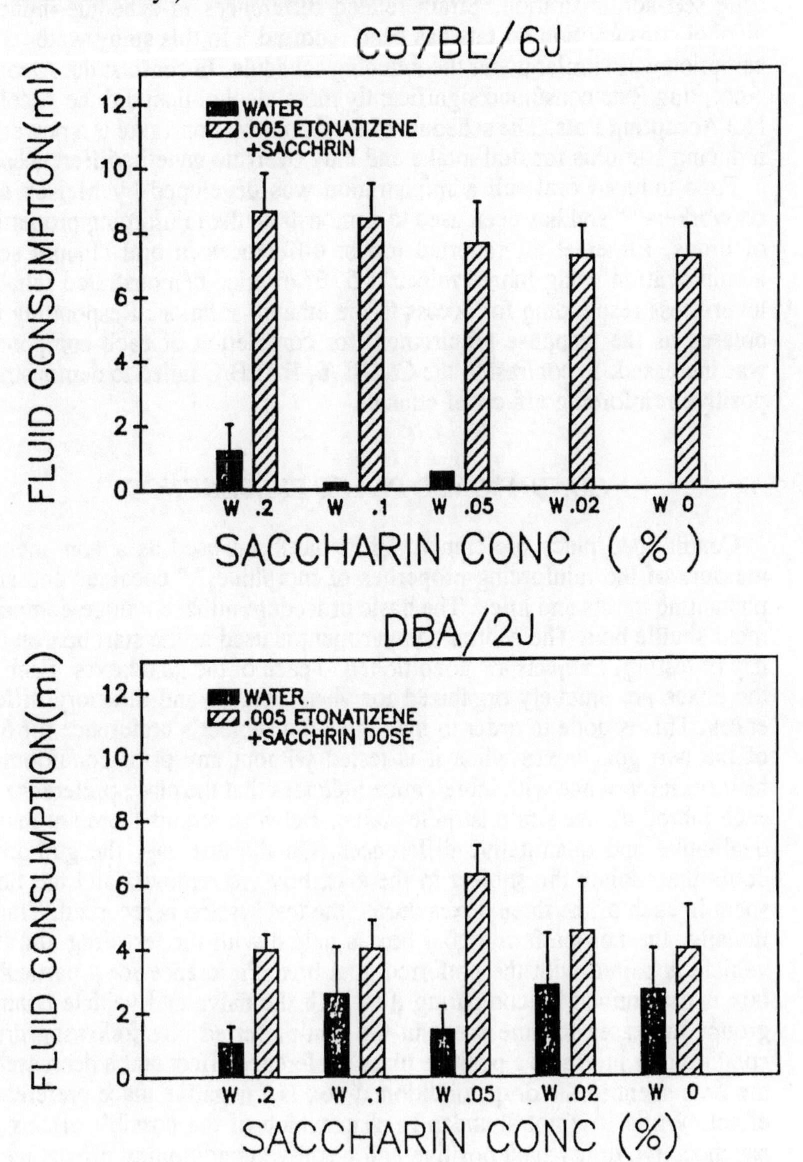

Tang[30] demonstrated that schedule induced polydypsia resulted in substantial intake of cocaine in rats. Schedule-induced polydypsia has not been systemically employed in the study of genetic determinants differences in drug self-administration. Strain related differences in schedule-induced alcohol consumption by rats has been reported.[31] In this study water consumption was similar under the inducing schedule. In contrast the Alcohol Accepting Rats consumed significantly more alcohol than did the Alcohol Not Accepting Rats. The schedule of food presentation value is a powerful inducing stimulus for oral intake and may override genetic differences.

Food-induced oral self-administration was developed by Meisch and co-workers[31-34] and has been used to demonstrate the reinforcing properties of drugs. Elmer et al. reported robust differences in oral ethanol self-administration using inbred mice.[34] C57BL/6 mice demonstrated reliable lever-press responding for access to the ethanol solution. Responding increased as the response requirement for completion of each component was increased. In contrast to the C57BL/6, BALB/C failed to demonstrate positive reinforcing effects of ethanol.

CONDITIONED PLACE PREFERENCE

Conditioned place preference (CPP) has been used as a non-operant measure of the reinforcing properties of morphine,[36,37] cocaine[39] and amphetamine in rats and mice. The basic procedure utilized a three-compartment shuttle box. The central compartment is used as the start box on the day of testing. Subjects are conditioned to each of the goal boxes. Each of the boxes are uniquely organized for visual, tactile and olfactory differences. This is done in order to maximize the subject's preference for one of the two goal boxes when it is tested without any prior conditioning history. Experience with inbred mice indicates that the place preference of each inbred mouse strain is quite stable. Between strains there are major qualitative and quantitative differences. On the test day, the guillotine doors that isolate the subject in the start box are removed and the time spent in each of the three boxes during the test session is recorded. Traditionally, the non-preferred goal box is paired with the test drug and the vehicle is paired with the preferred goal box. Preference for a particular box is determined by comparing it to both the naive and vehicle control group. Increases in time spent in the non-preferred box following drug conditioning indicates a positive place preference effect and a decrease in the time spent in the drug conditioned box is a negative place preference effect. While it is not abundantly clear which of the possible effects of psychoactive drugs such positive and negative conditioning effects identify, it is clear that drugs that have been demonstrated to function as positive reinforcers in operant evaluations, also demonstrate positive place preference effects.

In an initial evaluation of the CPP effects of etonitazene and its relationship to the above described differences in oral self-administration, C57BL and DBA mice were given a one day condition exposure and then tested for place preference on the next day. No injections (drug or vehicle) were given on the day of testing. Similar to the pattern of oral self-administration discussed above, the C57BL mice demonstrated a robust and dose-related positive place preference (Figure 3). In contrast to the C57BL mice, DBA mice demonstrated neither a positive nor a negative preference after conditioning. The fact that etonitazene failed to demonstrate negative place preference effects may indicate that the inherent differences in the self-administration of etonitazene in the two strains is the result of differences in the systems that mediate the positive reinforcing effects and not due to an increase in the negative reinforcement systems.

INTRAVENOUS SELF-ADMINISTRATION

As was discussed for oral self-administration, the characterization of drugs as reinforcing stimuli has relied on the demonstration of the positive reinforcing effects of response contingent intravenous drug delivery. Following surgical implantation of an intravenous catheter, subjects are given access to intravenous drug injections. The simplest situation for the characterization of the reinforcing effects of a drug is one in which the drug is infused following each operant response. Operant responses are experimentally defined and may be a lever press,[6] interruption of photocell beam by a nose poke[10] or some other operationally defined behavior.[18] The important factor in these experiments is the contingent relationship between the antecedent behavior (operant response) and the stimulus presentation (drug injection). In an initial demonstration of this procedure in inbred mice, the reinforcing effects of morphine was studied in a group of BALB/cBy mice. Each nose poke response resulted in the intravenous delivery of 0.5 mg/kg/injection of morphine on the drug test day and delivery of saline on the baseline control test day (Figure 4). While there were intersubject differences in the extent of morphine self-administration, all mice demonstrated a substantially greater number of morphine injections during at least one of the hourly components of the 6 hour session, compared to saline injections baseline. The magnitude of the self-administration was quite dramatic. In fact, morphine intake as high as 150-170 mg/kg occurred.

FIGURE 3. Inherent differences in conditioned place preference effects of etonitazene in C57BL/2J mice. Each bar represents the results of 6 mice tested one day after conditioning to saline in the black compartment and etonitazene in the white compartment. Mice were used only once.

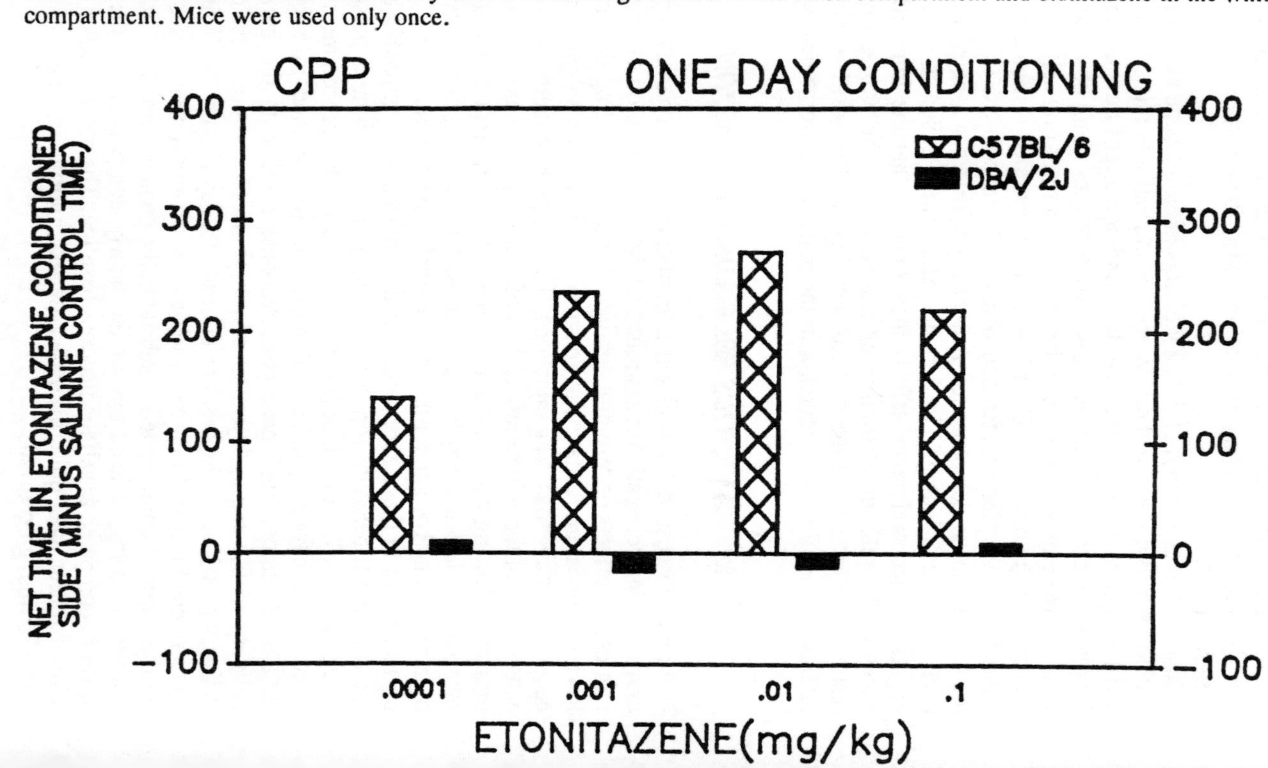

FIGURE 4. Intravenous self-administration morphine by BALB/cByJ mice. The open symbols represent saline injections for individual mice during the baseline control day (the day immediately prior to before morphine availability). Solid symbols represent the number of morphine injections during successive hours of the 6 hour session for each of the subjects.

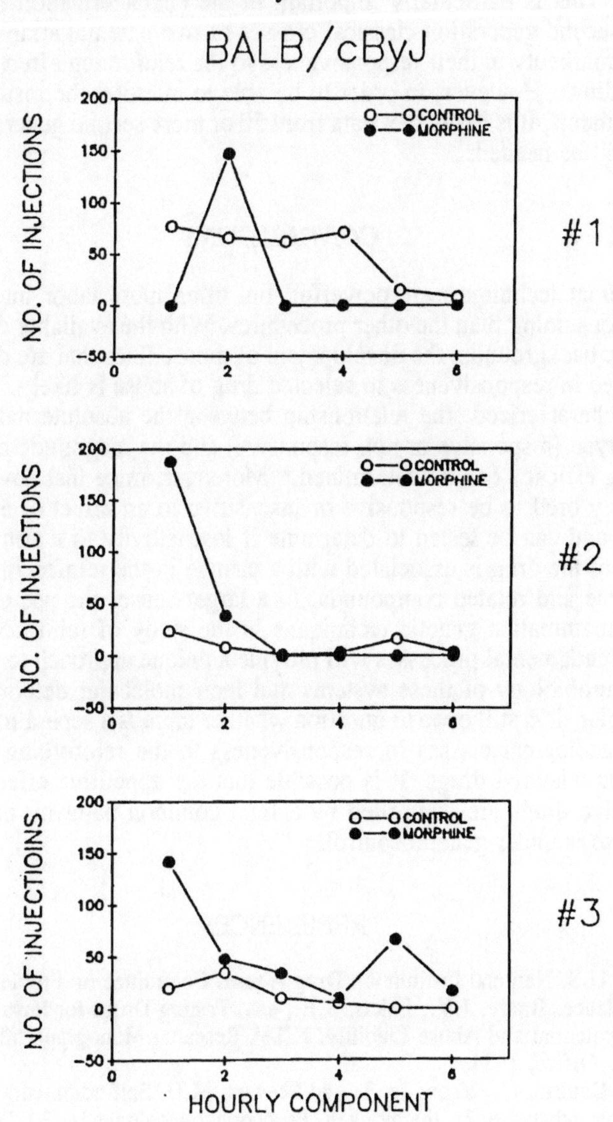

The defining characteristic of drugs that function as reinforcers is that they reliably maintain responding above baseline values. Because the baseline value in these studies is determined for each subject prior to the first access to drug injections, it is possible to characterize individual differences. This is particularly important in the characterization of progeny from second generation classical crosses of two parental strains that may differ markedly in their responsiveness to the reinforcing effects of prototypic drugs. However, in order to be able to interpret the results of such experiments, it is likely that data from 50 or more second generation progeny will be needed.

CONCLUSIONS

Operant techniques are powerful, but often more labor intensive and time consuming than the other procedures. With the available diversity of genetic backgrounds, the development of mouse lines that are deficient or enriched in responsiveness to selected drug of abuse is likely.[24] Once initially characterized, the relationship between the absolute nature of the phenotype (responsive or non-responsive) and the magnitude of the reinforcing efficacy can be determined.[39] Moreover, mice that have been selectively bred to be responsive or insensitive to an effect of a particular compound can be tested to determine if insensitivity to a non-appetitive effect of the drug is associated with a change in the reinforcing effect of the same and related compounds. In a larger sense, the use of sophisticated mammalian genetic techniques in the study of reinforcement and other fundamental processes will provide a unique approach to describing the neurobiology of these systems and their molecular determinants. In particular, it is still open to question whether there is a separation between pharmacological classes in responsiveness to the reinforcing effects of self-administered drugs. It is possible that the appetitive effects of psychoactive drugs are controlled by a final common pathway in the brain that also is under genetic control.

REFERENCES

1. U.S. National Institute on Drug Abuse. Committee on Problems of Drug Dependence. Brady, J.V., Lukas, S.E., eds. Testing Drugs for Physical Dependence Potential and Abuse Liability. NIDA Research Monograph 52. US Govt. Printing Office, 1984.

2. Deneau, G., Yanagita, T. and Seevers. M.H. Self-administration of psychoactive substances by the monkey. Psychopharmacologia 16: 30-48, 1969.

3. Hollister, L.E. Present use of hallucinogens. In: Saletu, B., Berner, P., Hollister, L. E., eds. Neuropyschopharmacology Proceeding of the llth Congress of CINP. Oxford, England, Pergamon Press. 1979: 182-192.

4. Ford, R.D. and Balster, R.L. Reinforcing properties of intravenous procaine in rhesus monkeys. Pharmacol. Biochem. Behav. 1977; 6: 289-296.

5. Kalant, H., LeBlanc. A.E., Gibbins, R.J. Tolerance to and dependence on some non-opiate psychotropic drugs. Pharmacol. Rev. 23: 135-191, 1971.

6. Woods, J.H. and Schuster, C.R. Opiates as reinforcing stimuli. In: Thompson, T., Pickens, R., eds. Stimulus Properties of Drugs. Appleton-Century-Crofts, New York 1971: 163-175.

7. Balster, R.L. and Johansen, C.E. The Pharmacology of Cocaine Related to its Abuse. Pharmacol. Rev. 41: 3-52, 1989.

8. Castellano, C. and Oliverio, A. A genetic analysis of morphine induced running and analgesia in the mouse. Psychopharmacologia (Berlin) 41: 197-200, 1975.

9. Brase, D.H., Loh, H.H. and Way, E.L. Comparison of the effects of morphine on locomotor activity, analgesia and primary and protracted physical dependence in six mouse strains. J. Pharmacol. Exp. Ther. 201: 368-373, 1977.

10. Crabbe, J.C. and Belknap, J.K. Pharmacogenetic tools in the study of drug tolerance and dependence. Subs. Alcohol Act. 1: 385-413. 1980.

11. Marks, M.J.. Romm, E., Bealer, S. and Collins, A.C. A test battery for measuring nicotine effects in mice. Pharmacol. Biochem. Behav. 23: 325-330, 1985.

12. Logan, L., Seale, T.W., Cao, W. and Carney, J.M. Effects of chronic amphetamine in BALB/cByJ mice, a strain that is not stimulated by the acute administration of amphetamine. Pharmacol. Biochem. Behav. 33: 99-105, 1989.

13. Carney, J.M., Seale, T.W., Logan, L., McMaster, S. Sensitivity of inbred mice to methylxanthines is not determined by plasma xanthine concentrations. Neuro. Letters 56: 27-31, 1985.

14. Seale, T.W., Roderick, T.H., Johnson, P., Logan, Rennert, O.M., and Carney, J.M. Complex genetic determinants of susceptibility to methylxanthine-induced locomotor activity changes. Pharmacol. Biochem. Behav. 24: 1333-1341, 1986.

15. Snyder, S.H., Katims, J.J., Annau, Z., Bruns. R.F. and Daly, J.W. Andenosine receptors and behavioral actions of methylxanthines. Proc. Natl. Acad. Sci. 78: 3260-3264. 1981.

16. Kelleher, R.T. and Morse, W. Determinants of the specificity of the behavioral effects of drugs. Ergeb. Physiol. Chem. Exp. Pharmak. 60: 1-56, 1968.

17. Kelleher, R.T. Characteristics of behavior controlled by scheduled injections of drugs. Pharmacol. Rev. 27: 307-323, 1976.

18. Wenger, G.R. and Dews, P.B. The effects of phencyclidine, ketamine, d-amphetamine and pentabarbital on schedule-controlled responding in the mouse. J. Pharmacol. Exp. Ther. 196: 616-624, 1976.

19. Wenger, G. Some quantitative behavioral pharmacology in the mouse. In:

Thompson, T. and Dews, P.B., eds. Advances in Behavioral Pharmacology, Vol. 2. New York, Academic Press, 1979: 1-38.

20. Hebb, D. and Levine, T. Effects of caffeine on DRL performance in the mouse. Pharmacol. Biochem. Behav. 9:7-10, 1978.

21. Katz, J.L. Interactions of clonidine and naloxone on schedule-controlled behavior in opioid naive mice. Psychopharmacology 98: 445-447, 1989.

22. Gwynn, G. and Domino, E.F. Genotype dependent behavioral sensitivity to *mu* and *kappa* opiate agonists: I. Acute and chronic effects on mouse locomotor activity. J. Pharmacol. Exp. Ther 231: 306-311, 1989.

23. Oliverio, A. and Costellano, C. Genotype-dependent sensitivity and tolerance to morphine and heroin: Dissociation between opiate induced running and analgesics in the mouse. Pyschopharmacologia 39: 13-22, 1974.

24. Moskowitz, A.S., Terman, G.W., Carter, K.R., Morgan, M.J., Liebeskind, J.C. Analgesic, locomotor, and lethal effects of morphine in the mouse: Strain comparisons. Brain Res. 361: 46-51, 1985.

25. Horowitz, G.P., Whitney, G., Smith, J.C., Stephan, F.K. Morphine ingestion: Genetic control in mice. Psychopharmacologia 52: 119-122, 1977.

26. Falk, J.L. Production of polydypsia in normal rats by intermittent food schedule. Science 133: 195-196, 1961.

27. Falk, J.L. Analysis of water and NaCl solution acceptance by schedule-induced polydypsia. J. Exp. Anal. Behav. 9: 11-118, 1966.

28. Falk, J.L. and Tang, M. Schedule-induction of drug intake: Differential responsiveness to agents with abuse potential. J. Pharmacol. Exp. Ther. 249: 143-148, 1989.

29. McMillan, D.C. and Leander, J.D. Schedule-induced oral self-administration of etonitazene. Pharmacol. Biochem. Behav. 4: 137-141, 1976.

30. Falk, J.L. and Teng, M. Schedule-induced chlordiazepoxide intake: differential effects of cocaine and ethanol histories. Pharmacol. Biochem. Behav. 33: 393-396, 1989.

31. Ritz. M.C. George, F.R., and Meisch, R.A. Ethanol Self-administration in ALKO Rats: I. Effects of selection and concentration. Alcohol 6: 227-233, 1989.

32. Meisch, R.A. and Beardsley, P. Ethanol as a reinforcer in rats: Effects of concurrent access to water and alternate positions of ethanol and water. Psychopharmacologia 43: 19-23, 1975.

33. Elmer, G.E., Meisch, R.A., Goldberg, S.R., George, F.R. Fixed ratio schedules of oral ethanol self-administration in inbred strains of mice. Psychopharm. 96: 431-436, 1988.

34. Ritz, M.C., George, F.R., DeFiebre, C.M., Meisch, R.A. Genetic differences in the establishment of ethanol as a reinforcer. Pharmacol. Biochem. Behav. 24: 3260-3264, 1986.

35. Elmer, G.I., Meisch, R.A. and George, F.R. Oral ethanol reinforced behavior in inbred mice. Pharmacol. Biochem. Behav. 24: 1417-1422, 1986.

36. Bardo, M.J., Miller, J.S., Neisewander, J.L. Conditioned place prefer-

ence with morphine: The effect of extinction training on the reinforcing CR. Pharmacol. Biochem. Behav. 1984; 21: 545-550.

37. Mucha, R.F. and Iversen, S.D. Reinforcing properties of morphine and naloxone revealed by conditioned place preferences: A procedural examination. Psychopharm. 82: 241-247, 1984.

38. Nomickos, G.G. and Spyraki, C. Cocaine-induced place conditioning: Importance of the route of administration and other procedural variables. Psychopharm. 94: 119-125, 1988.

39. Spyraki, C., Fibiger, H.C. and Phillips, A.G. Dopamine substrates of amphetamine-induced place preference conditioning. Brain Res. 253:13-16, 1982.

40. Crabbe, J.C. Sensitivity to ethanol in inbred mice: Genotypic correlations among several behavioral responses. Behav. Neurosci. 97: 280-289, 1983.

Establishment of Drug Discrimination and Drug Reinforcement in Different Animal Strains: Some Methodological Issues

Richard A. Meisch, MD, PhD

SUMMARY. The study of drug reinforcement and drug discrimination in different animal strains raises some methodological issues. Potential problems are discussed, and some possible solutions are mentioned. A distinction is made between establishment of drug reinforced behavior and the maintenance of drug reinforced behavior. A similar distinction holds for the establishment and maintenance of drug discriminations. Strain differences may arise during either the establishment or maintenance phases. Interpretation of findings of strain differences is also discussed. Lastly, a distinction is made between drug self-administration and drug reinforcement.

Study of the genetics of drug reinforcement and drug discrimination presents some methodological problems. Both drug reinforcement and drug discrimination involve conditioned behavior (i.e., learned behavior). A comparison between animal strains of conditioned behavior requires that the conditioning be successfully accomplished in each strain.

In behavioral pharmacology, within-subject designs are almost exclu-

---

Richard A. Meisch is affiliated with the Department of Psychiatry and Behavioral Sciences, and Department of Pharmacology, University of Texas Health Science Center at Houston.

Reprint requests may be addressed to Richard A. Meisch, Psychiatry/UTHSC-H, 1300 Moursund, Houston, TX 77030-3406.

The author thanks Dr. Gregory A. Lemaire for his helpful comments on the manuscript.

Preparation of this manuscript was supported by Grant DA00944 from the National Institute on Drug Abuse, USPHS.

sively used. Because the emphasis is usually on establishing comparable performances across subjects and not on testing subjects under identical values of independent variables, somewhat different conditions are often employed with different subjects. For example, if one method of establishing a drug as a reinforcer does not work, then a second method is tried. In one study with rhesus monkeys, intravenous ethanol self-administration was examined.[6] Some of the monkeys initiated responding when each lever press resulted in an infusion of 0.1 or 0.2 gm/kg of ethanol; other monkeys did not initiate responding. For these other monkeys their ethanol solution was replaced with either methohexital (0.5 mg/kg) or cocaine (0.5 mg/kg). Responding was initiated and maintained by infusion of these drugs. Subsequently the monkeys were switched back to ethanol and all animals, regardless of their acquisition procedure, self-injected the ethanol solutions in similar patterns and amounts (Winger and Woods, 1973). This type of strategy is common in behavioral pharmacology.

In behavior genetics the situation is different. Between-subject designs (i.e., group designs) are used, and the emphasis is on holding experimental conditions, including past experience, constant so that differences between groups reflect differences in genotype and not differences in environmental factors.

Since the two disciplines typically employ different experimental strategies, problems arise when combining the two areas. In behavioral pharmacology, most studies concern conditioned behavior. In particular, the study of drugs as reinforcers and as discriminative stimuli involves conditioning. A positive reinforcer is defined as an event which, when presented contingent upon a response, increases the subsequent probability of the response, and a discriminative stimulus is a stimulus in the presence of which a response is reinforced and in the absence of which it is not reinforced.[1] The study of conditioned behavior is often more complicated than study of unconditioned behavior. One complexity is that conditioned behavior has phases such as acquisition, maintenance, and extinction.[4] Behavior that has been learned is usually in a steady state. For example, the behavior of an experienced bicycle rider is very different from that of one who is learning to ride. In contrast to the steady-state maintenance phase, behavior that is developing or being learned is said to be in a transition phase (i.e., the pattern of the behavior often undergoes change from one occurrence to the next). What do these distinctions have to do with the study of genetic factors in drug discrimination and drug reinforcement? The answer is that these distinctions must be explicitly set forth before several problems can be adequately discussed.

If one is to compare the reinforcing or discriminative effects of drugs across several strains, then one must condition the behavior of these animals. Specifically, one must first *establish* the drug as a reinforcer or as a discriminative stimulus. *The problem is that conditions or procedures which may be effective in establishing the drug as a reinforcer (or discriminative stimulus) in one strain may not be effective in another strain.* That is, genetic differences may result in problems in the acquisition phase such that in a particular strain it is difficult to obtain drug reinforced or drug discrimination behavior. So what does one do? Several strategies will be suggested. More than one strategy may need to be used to arrive at a satisfactory solution.

ESTABLISHMENT OF DRUGS AS REINFORCERS OR DISCRIMINATIVE STIMULI

1. Conservative Training

One strategy is to be conservative and use procedures that are highly likely to work with all animals tested. For example, in attempting to establish ethanol as a reinforcer for both Lewis and Fischer 344 rats, extended training procedures were employed to ensure that both groups mastered the behaviors of lever pressing and drinking from the liquid delivery system.[5] During the acquisition phase a low ethanol concentration (1% w/v) was used, and the concentration of ethanol was gradually increased in steps to 5.7%. The objective was to avoid employing conditions that might lead to ethanol developing as a reinforcer for only one of the strains. A conservative approach also allows the tentative conclusion that if a drug is not established as a reinforcer for a particular strain, then the failure is more likely to be a reflection of genotype rather than of an inadequate training procedure. The major disadvantage of a conservative approach is the time required to implement it.

2. Separate Exploratory Parametric Studies

A second approach is to conduct separate sets of exploratory studies with each strain, and not attempt to treat each strain in an identical manner. Ideally the results of such studies would lead to the identification of test conditions that are appropriate for each strain. The aim is to devise a common procedure to use across strains, even though it may be a compromise in not being maximally effective with any strain. In follow-up studies one would then use identical training protocols with each strain. Potential drawbacks to this approach again include the time required and the possibility that it may not be possible to identify identical test conditions that result in the development of drugs as discriminative stimuli or reinforcers for all strains under study.

3. Informed Guess Based on Existing Data

A third possibility is to use existing data on the effects of the drug in the different strains that are to be studied. For example, the doses that result in changes in food-reinforced behavior or changes in open field activity may be known. These data may permit the selection of appropriate doses to use in drug discrimination training. This approach also has limitations. An extensive behavioral data base for a drug may not exist, or if it does, the information may not be of use in selecting doses for use in studies of drug discrimination or drug reinforced behavior. As with the first two approaches this approach lacks a guarantee of success.

4. Different Procedures

A fourth approach is one that has a serious flaw and should only be used as a last resort. This approach is to use different training procedures with each strain if, and only if, success cannot be achieved by use of an identical procedure with all strains. The rationale is simple: one cannot compare conditioned behavior in different strains unless the conditioned behavior is present in those strains. The drawback to using different training procedures is that subsequent differences between two strains may be due at least in part to different experimental histories and not to different genotypes.

It is important to note that if a training procedure works with one strain but not with another, then one has found a difference between strains. A reasonable next step if a strain difference is found would be to experimentally determine the basis of the difference.

5. More Than One of the Above

A fifth procedure may be termed "some or all of the above." In other words a satisfactory answer may come only by employing more than one strategy.

MAINTENANCE OF DRUG REINFORCED BEHAVIOR OR DRUG DISCRIMINATION BEHAVIOR

Once one has successfully established a drug as a reinforcer or discriminative stimulus for two or more strains, it becomes possible to examine differences and similarities among strains. That there will probably be differences, as well as similarities, will not surprise behavior geneticists. The point to be made is that it is important to study behavior over a range of conditions. For example, Figure 1 shows the number of lever presses as a function of ethanol concentration for two strains, Lewis and Fischer 344 rats, under conditions where a lever press was required to produce access to small volumes of ethanol.

Examining a range of concentrations provided a systematic replication of differences between strains and also avoided the problem of picking values that were optimal for one strain but not for another (Suzuki et al., 1988). There is an additional reason for looking over a range of values of the independent variables. In another experiment with Lewis and Fischer 344 rats, ethanol maintained higher rates of responding in the Lewis than in the Fischer rats over a range of fixed-ratio values (Suzuki et al., 1988). However, with other pairs of strains one might see functions such as these cross over: Assume that at FR 1 responding by rats of Strain A is lower than that of rats of Strain B, as illustrated in Figure 2. However, at higher fixed-ratio sizes Strain A rats might display higher rates than those displayed by Strain B rats. Were one to examine only a single FR value, one might draw misleading conclusions.

INTERPRETATION AND EXPLANATION OF STRAIN DIFFERENCES IN BEHAVIOR CONTROLLED BY DRUG REINFORCERS OR DRUG DISCRIMINATIVE STIMULI

Once strain differences in behavior controlled by drug reinforcers or drug discriminative stimuli have been observed, interpreting or explaining such differences becomes the focus of interest. Several approaches are possible.

One approach is to use classical genetic methods such as crossbreeding experiments. A second is to analyze pharmacokinetic and pharmacodynamic differences. A third is to conduct further behavioral studies. For example, in the Suzuki et al. study[5] there were differences between Lewis and Fischer 344 rats in ethanol reinforced fixed-ratio performance. It is possible that these differences are not specific to ethanol as a reinforcer. If

FIGURE 1. Responses as a function of ethanol concentration for Lewis and Fischer 344 rats. Each point is a mean of 20 sessions (4 rats x 5 sessions each). Vertical lines are the standard errors of the mean (n = 4). Circles represent results obtained with the Lewis strain, and squares represent results obtained with the Fischer 344 strain. Closed and open symbols represent the ascending and descending ethanol concentration series, respectively. This figure is adapted from Panel A of Figure 3 in Suzuki et al., 1988.

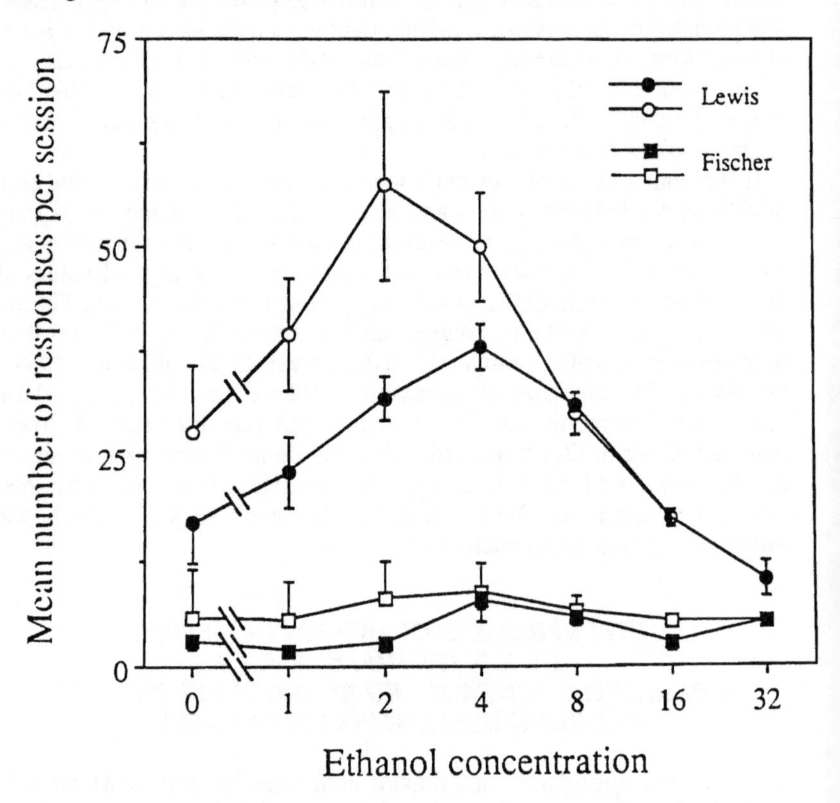

other reinforcers such as saccharin solutions had been studied, similar differences might have been found. Further behavioral studies are thus suggested. Another example is that direct rate altering effects of drugs also may result in differences in drug reinforced performance. In one strain self-administration of large amounts of barbiturate may lead to marked decreases in response rate because of effects on motor performance. In a different strain similar barbiturate intakes may have minor effects on motor function. Different rates of barbiturate reinforced behavior would probably occur in the two strains. One way to control for such

FIGURE 2. Response rate as a function of fixed-ratio size for two rat strains: A and B. Note that these are hypothetical data.

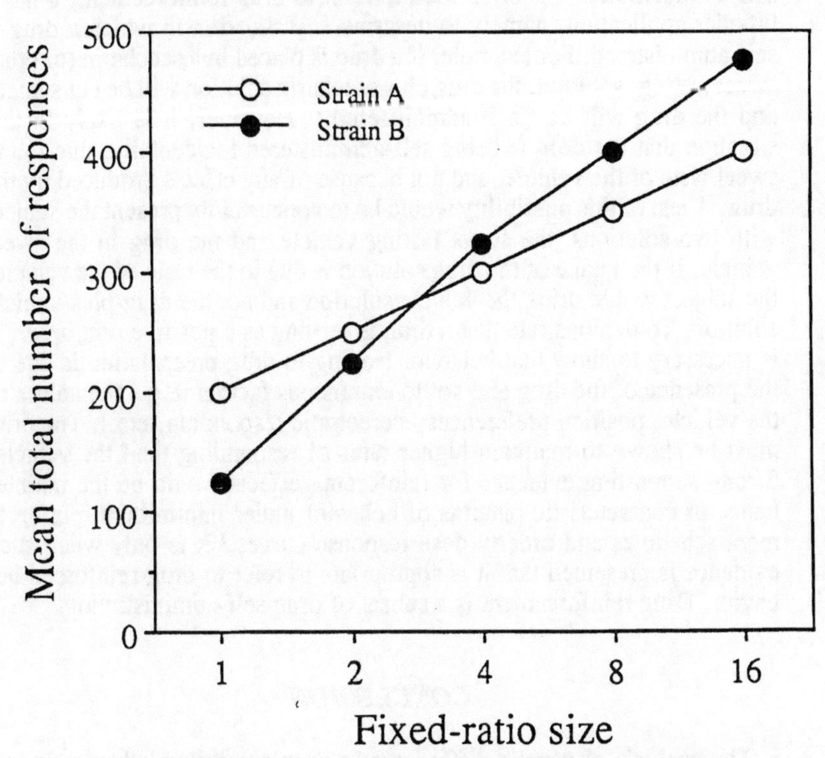

differences in drug effects on motor function is to make the drug available only at the end of an experimental session. This procedure was developed by Goldberg and colleagues,[2] and it permits one to examine reinforcing effects in the absence of other drug effects. The important point is that it is possible and highly desirable to investigate the variables contributing to strain differences at the behavioral level as well as at other levels of analysis (e.g., the cellular and molecular levels).

THE DISTINCTION BETWEEN DRUG SELF-ADMINISTRATION AND DRUG REINFORCED BEHAVIOR

A final methodological point is that the terms "drug self-administration" and "drug reinforced behavior" are often confused, and this is due in part to researchers using these phrases synonymously. Although "drug self-administration" is often used to refer to drug reinforcement, it has a broader application, namely to describe any situation in which a drug is self-administered. For example, if a drug is placed in a saccharin (or other sweet tasting) solution, the drug plus saccharin solution will be consumed, and the drug will be "self-administered." However, it is likely in this situation that the drug is being self-administered incidentally, due to the sweet taste of the vehicle, and not because of any effects produced by the drug. A test of this possibility would be to concurrently present the subject with two solutions: the sweet tasting vehicle and the drug in the sweet vehicle. If the intake of the drug solution is due to the taste of the vehicle, the subject would drink the vehicle solution and not the drug-plus-vehicle solution. To demonstrate that a drug is serving as a positive *reinforcer*, it is necessary to show that behavior leading to drug presentation is due to the presence of the drug and not to extraneous factors (e.g., the nature of the vehicle, position preferences, stereotypic responding, etc.). The drug must be shown to maintain higher rates of responding than the vehicle. Strong supporting evidence for reinforcing effects would be the maintenance of characteristic patterns of behavior under intermittent reinforcement schedules and orderly dose response curves.[3] It is only when such evidence is presented that it is appropriate to refer to drug-reinforced behavior. Drug reinforcement is a subset of drug self-administration.

CONCLUSION

The analysis of genetic differences in drug controlled behavior is just beginning. This analysis will require resolution of some methodological problems. The strategies mentioned above are suggestions of possible ways to proceed. One measure of progress in this area will be the development and validation of appropriate experimental methods.

REFERENCES

1. Ferster CB, Skinner BF. Schedules of reinforcement. Englewood Cliffs, New Jersey: Prentice-Hall, 1957.

2. Goldberg SR, Morse WH, Goldberg DM. Behavior maintained under a second-order schedule by intramuscular injection of morphine or cocaine in rhesus monkeys. J Pharmacol Exp Ther 1976; 199:278-286.

3. Meisch RA, Carroll ME. Oral drug self-administration: Drugs as reinforcers. In: Bozarth MA, ed. Methods of assessing the reinforcing properties of abused drugs. New York: Springer-Verlag, 1989:143-160.

4. Sidman M. Tactics of scientific research. New York: Basic Books, Inc., 1960.

5. Suzuki T, George FR, Meisch RA. Differential establishment and maintenance of oral ethanol reinforced behavior in Lewis and Fischer 344 inbred rat strains. J Pharmacol Exp Ther 1988; 245:164-170.

6. Winger GD, Woods JH. The reinforcing property of ethanol in the rhesus monkey: I. Initiation, maintenance and termination of intravenous ethanol-reinforced responding. Ann NY Acad Sci 1973; 215:162-175.

Biochemical Genetic Differences in Vulnerability to Drug Effects: Is Statistically Significant Always Physiologically Important and Vice Versa?

Mary C. Ritz, PhD

SUMMARY. The goal of biochemical genetic experiments, which are designed to better understand vulnerability to drug effects, is to determine variation in biochemical traits which can account for variation in behavioral and physiological effects of drugs. Biochemical genetic experiments commonly span several distinct scientific disciplines and many different methodologies, both behavioral and biochemical. In most cases, biochemical genetic experiments involve at least three different levels of analysis, including sophisticated mathematical models of genetic inheritance, many behavioral paradigms used to assess various drug-related phenotypes, and a variety of biochemical methodologies used to determine biochemical correlates. Both the multidisciplinary nature of this scientific endeavor and the traditional uses of the scientific methods which are now being applied to pharmacogenetic experiments necessitate careful consideration of many often conflicting theoretical perspectives in the process of interpretation of experimental results. Several scientific considerations are discussed which emphasize the presentation of the results of pharmacogenetic studies within the context of expectations concerning genetic variance as well as traditional uses and assumptions related to methodology.

Mary C. Ritz is affiliated with the Behavioral Pharmacology and Genetics Laboratory, National Institute on Drug Abuse, Baltimore, MD 21224.

Address correspondence to: Dr. Mary C. Ritz, NIDA Addiction Research Center, 4940 Eastern Avenue, Baltimore, MD 21224.

INTRODUCTION

The scientific field of behavior genetics encompasses the study of variation in behavior among individuals, and the degree to which genetic and environmental factors influence this variation. Pharmacogenetics is a related field concerned with the effects of genetic factors on drug effects. Behavioral pharmacogenetic studies using both human and animal populations have demonstrated that sensitivity to drugs, tolerance to drugs and drug-reinforced behavior are complex phenomena mediated by genetic and environmental factors and by critical interactions between these factors. Most recently, the evidence is increasing for genetic vulnerability to most drug effects in certain individuals or populations. Recognition of these differences suggests the influence of inherited biological factors which predispose individuals to greater or lesser drug effects. Further, understanding how drugs interact with the central nervous system to produce either reinforcing or toxic effects, increases the probability that the potentially harmful effects of these compounds may be blocked, or at least attenuated, by the development of more effective prevention and treatment programs.

The goal of biochemical pharmacogenetic experiments, which are designed to better understand vulnerability to drug effects, is to determine variation in biochemical traits which can account for variation in behavioral and physiological effects of drugs. Most biochemical genetic studies focus at the level of the neuron, at neurotransmitters, peptides, receptors and enzymes. Gene expression, localization and interactions between neuronal systems have also increasingly become targets of analysis. The primary task of the biochemical pharmacogeneticist is that of describing variation in biochemical events that might be associated with individual differences and train differences in drug response. This paper is an attempt to raise practical questions and issues, inherent in this scientific endeavor, which must be considered in order to effectively persuade the scientific community, and perhaps the general public, of proposed mechanisms of genetic vulnerability.

WHEN DOES A BIOCHEMICAL GENETIC DIFFERENCE MAKE A DIFFERENCE?

This question arises predominately for two reasons. First, biochemical pharmacogenetics as a distinct scientific discipline is inherently a multidisciplinary endeavor. Biochemical genetic experiments commonly incorporate several distinct scientific disciplines and many different methodologies, both behavioral and biochemical. In most cases, biochemical genetic experiments involve at least three different levels of analysis. At one level, sophisticated mathematical models of genetic inheritance are commonly utilized. These models are valuable for comparing the expected occurrence of a phenotype, given a particular mode of inheritance, with the actual observed occurrence of the phenotype. They also allow us to estimate the approximate number of genes which appear to influence a particular drug effect. At yet another level of analysis, a variety of behavioral paradigms are used to assess sensitivity to drugs, tolerance for drugs and dependence on drugs. These effects as well as the discriminative and reinforcing, or potentially addictive, effects can be assessed in operant self-administration studies. In a third level of analysis, the cellular mechanisms associated with a behavioral or physiological drug response are examined using various biochemical methodologies. The latter are rapidly and constantly increasing in complexity and number. In summary, pharmacogenetic analyses involve several theoretical models, each having its specialized language and definitions which must be accurately and effectively used in the interpretation and discussion of experimental results.

Thus, present day biochemical pharmacogenetic studies encompass the fields of experimental psychology, pharmacology, neuroscience, immunology and molecular genetics. A biochemical pharmacogeneticist is, in effect, a nearly proverbial "jack-of-all-traits," a renaissance person. Accordingly, the task of an effective biochemical pharmacogeneticist has become increasingly complex. Though scientists in other fields have often become increasingly specialized, the biochemical geneticist has necessarily become increasingly multidisciplinary in the effort to bridge the theoretical and philosophical gaps between behaviorists, biochemists and geneticists.

The second reason for such a query is that expectations concerning the type of biochemical trait and the magnitude of difference in that trait that might likely be associated with genetic differences in a drug response have not been well established to date. In fact, the experts who have developed both behavioral and biochemical methodologies which are utilized by biochemical geneticists are not in absolute agreement that genetic differences in biochemical traits are expected or important for determining drug effects. For example, in the field of behavioral pharmacology, operant methodologies have typically been used to study the reinforcing effects of drugs and the environmental cues which influence drug self-administration behavior in both animal and human experimental paradigms. It is not surprising, since drug use and abuse have traditionally been treated predominantly as psychosocial problems, that it has often been assumed that environmental factors, not inherited traits, are primarily responsible for drug-seeking behavior. In general, drugs which are typically abused by human beings generally serve as reinforcers in animal subjects from several species.[1] Thus, it has been commonly assumed that, with few exceptions, animal subjects given the appropriate training/environmental cues and drug history would self-administer drugs which had previously been shown to serve as reinforcers. Experimental results were often described for individual animals due to large individual differences in response patterns. In addition, animal subjects for which a drug did not serve as a reinforcer were replaced by others which emitted drug-seeking behaviorism, thus eliminating abstainers from the subject pool. Individual differences between subjects, however, were not generally described in terms of inherited traits.

Similarly, neuroscientists developed receptor binding techniques in order to measure and localize brain effector proteins which specifically bound to various endogenous neurotransmitters, thus enabling the chemical transmission or modification of electrical signals from one neuron to the next. For these purposes, subclassifications of receptors have been described in terms of relatively gross differences in the affinity of a particular ligand for the receptors or unique pharmacology associated with a subclass of binding sites. In the past, the affinity of a particular ligand for a particular receptor subclass has been shown to be remarkably similar across strains and across species. Indeed, ligands and receptors have generally been thoroughly characterized initially, then subsequent research, though it may utilize different strains or species of animal subjects, quite effectively assumes affinity and receptor number to be equivalent. In general, neuroscientists who typically use receptor binding techniques answer the question "What magnitude of difference in K_D is worthy of further investigation?," with a response indicating that a 5-10 fold difference would be deemed important. The minimal receptor density differences required in order to warrant further investigation would generally thought to be 20-25 percent. These investigators typically have not often theorized about the finer genetic difference between strains of a single species with respect to a single subclass of receptor.

For yet another example, in the field of molecular genetics, there are many observations of sequence homology between different proteins designed to perform analogous functions. For example, many membrane-bound proteins, such as receptors or subunits of ion channel complexes, have nearly identical sequences associated with the process of incorporation into the cell membrane.[2,3,4,5,6] Other proteins requiring facilitating protein binding or cofactors, such as enzymes or receptors associated with second messenger systems, exhibit considerable sequence homology in regions associated with this function.[7] Indeed, this type of conservation and replication of genetic coding has become the basis of many attempts to retrieve previously undiscovered coding sequences for proteins which are presumed to perform similar or analogous biological functions. Molecular genetic studies have also shown that species variation is relatively low, enabling DNA segments derived from one species to serve as probes of the genetic material obtained from another species. Finally, even when variants in the coding sequences for a particular protein product are found, some functional assays are able to illustrate differences between proteins while other functional assays do not. For example, recent studies indicate that exchanges of heterogeneous alpha subunits of the $GABA_A$ receptor subtype are not associated with differential electrophysiological responses, while substitutions of these subunits for each other do alter the apparent sensitivity of the receptor to the neurotransmitter GABA.[7]

In essence, then, biochemical pharamcogeneticists often find themselves at the opposite end of one philosophical spectrum from those scientists who typically observe conservation of form in their daily experiments. Pharmacogeneticists often observe differences between animal strains for a variety of behavioral and physiological measures,[8,9] and experience teaches them that inherited differences in response to various drug effects is quite easy to illustrate. It follows that, biochemical geneticists might expect that biochemical variants should be observed, and would be expected to be associated with observed differences in behavioral effects of drugs. Given this disparity in scientific and philosophical bias, it is imperative that biochemical variants which are proposed to mediate specific drug responses be observed within the context of current and historical experience concerning both the trait of interest and the measure that is utilized.

STATISTICAL SIGNIFICANCE VS. BEHAVIORAL OR PHYSIOLOGICAL RELEVANCE

Two major questions must be considered in determining the relationship between an apparent difference in a biochemical trait and an observed genetic difference in response to a drug. First, "Are statistically significant differences necessarily physiologically or behaviorally important?" In some cases, deductions based on the results of previous studies may indeed provide important *a priori* evidence for an association between behavioral and biochemical phenotypes. Thus, new results concerning biochemical correlates can be placed in this context, which in turn provides confirmation of the proposed relationships. Theoretical problems arise, however, when several studies observe different statistically significant biochemical correlates associated with a drug effect. Indeed, taken together, these traits illogically might appear to account for in excess of 100% of the total variance in the behavioral phenotype. Since several variables may in act be correlated with each other, however, multivariate analyses could better indicate the relative proportion of influence of several biochemical correlates, while taking into account the covariance between factors. Furthermore, even when appropriate statistical measures are utilized and significant pharmacological or genetic correlations suggest biochemical mechanisms of drug responses, the limitations of the conclusions must be recognized. For example, it is possible that a pharmacological correlation showing the relationship between the potencies of several related drugs in producing a behavioral phenotype and their potencies in assays of a particular biochemical trait may illustrate a significant relationship. This result would suggest that the biochemical trait mediates, at least in part, the behavioral phenotype. This does not necessarily imply, however, that subsequent genetic correlations would show that the same biochemical mechanism could explain genetic differences in the drug response, especially if modulatory mechanisms indirectly impact upon this direct action of the drugs. In addition, distinct biochemical traits may differentially mediate the potency or efficacy of a drug in producing a particular effects. It is likely that both pharmacological and genetic correlations will be necessary to definitively show (1) which biochemical traits influence a drug response, (2) which of these traits, or others, influence sensitivity and maximal response to a drug, and (3) which traits mediate genetic differences in the drug response.

The second major question to be considered when evaluating the influence of a biochemical factor on a drug response is the flip side of the first, and asks "Are biochemical differences related to physiological or behavioral effects of drugs likely to be statistically significant differences?" Several considerations may influence the response to this query. It seems possible that current methods may not be adequately sensitive to distinguish what might be presumed to be small or discrete differences between individuals or strains of the same species. Alternatively, it is well known that the choice of subject genotype can influence the statistical significance of experimental results by dramatically limiting the range or variability in a particular measure. Thus, a correlational study may more effectively incorporate outbred animals rather than several inbred strains if these more effectively represent a true dispersion, rather than clusters, of phenotypic values. Additionally, in presenting the results of experiments using a particular methodology, one must consider the historical, traditional application of the measure. This process will enable one to predict methodological pitfalls and common questions associated with the conclusions of the research. For example, as discussed, the methodologies employed in the fields of neuroscience and molecular genetics are typically utilized to study gross differences between biological proteins, while biochemical genetic studies are grappling with the task of illustrating relatively fine distinctions between proteins which would nonetheless fall into the same functional subclassification. Yet another consideration might be that a biological protein can only be modified genetically to the extent that it retains its original function. Thus, the expected heritability and fitness value of the trait must be considered in order to estimate the expected magnitude of phenotypic variation. If the trait is vitally important for the viability of the organism, then it is not likely to vary greatly in normal, healthy subjects. Finally, it is imperative to consider information, if it exists, which predicts expected changes in a biochemical measure on the basis of known changes in genetic material or protein structure. It would be important to know, for example, the magnitude of change in receptor affinity which can be associated with a single amino acid change, or the effect of different genetic codes which, when translated, lead to a greater receptor density. It might be helpful to understand the effect of neuronal membrane composition on membrane fluidity or on the interaction of specific membrane lipids with the receptors. These pieces of data become extremely valuable for the interpretation of genetic correlations and other studies aimed at predicting biological vulnerability to a drug effect.

ILLUSTRATIVE RESEARCH EXAMPLES

Specific examples may more effectively illustrate several considerations which have been suggested as important in developing arguments concerning biochemical mechanisms which appear to mediate behavioral and physiological responses to drugs. For example, recently we proposed to identify the brain receptors which mediate the reinforcing properties of cocaine and other pharmacologically and chemically related drugs. In an effort to do so, the relationship between the potencies of these compounds in operant studies of drug self-administration behavior and their binding potencies at monoaminergic uptake sites and nearly 25 other neurotransmitter receptor sites was determined. The results of this research have shown that cocaine inhibition of striatal ^{3}H-mazindol binding to the dopamine transporter is significantly positively correlated with the reinforcing effects of cocaine-related drugs.[10]

This study illustrates the importance of a multivariate analysis for determining the relative proportion of influence of several biochemical parameters on a behavioral effect of a drug. In this particular study, each of the cocaine binding sites examined appeared to be linearly correlated with the drug effect. Moreover, drug potencies at one site were correlated with those at another. Figure 1 shows that the affinities of cocaine-related drugs for dopamine, norepinephrine and serotonin transporters individually and their potencies in cocaine self-administration studies are positively correl-

FIGURE 1. Pearson Correlation Matrix showing the relationships between the potency of cocaine and seven related compounds in self-administration studies (Behavior) and the potencies of these compounds to inhibit ligand binding at dopamine (DA), norepinephrine (NE) and serotonin (5-HT) transporters. Data taken from Ritz et al., 1987.

Pearson Correlation Matrix

	Behavior	DA	5-HT	NE
Behavior	1.00	0.94***	0.61	0.65
DA		1.00	0.77*	0.77*
5-HT			1.00	0.79**
NE				1.00

* P< .04
** P< .03
*** P< .002

ated. In addition, positive correlations are observed between the potencies of the cocaine-related drugs in inhibiting ligand binding to any two different transporter sites. Thus, though any of these sites studied individually would be observed to be linearly correlated with the reinforcing effects of cocaine, the multivariate analysis appropriately indicates that the dopamine transporter is the primary influence on self-administration. Indeed, this biochemical evidence is corroborated by many behavioral studies showing that dopaminergic mechanisms, but not noradrenergic and serotonergic mechanisms, have been implicated in the reinforcing effects of cocaine.[11,12,13,14,15,16,17,18,19]

Since cocaine inhibition of dopamine uptake appeared to account for over 90 percent of the variance in the reinforcing potency of cocaine and related drugs, subsequent experiments were designed to assess whether variation in the dopamine transporter might also explain genetic differences in oral cocaine self-administration. Recent studies have shown that cocaine, self-administered orally, serves as a strong reinforcer in Lewis rats, a marginal reinforcer in NBR rats and does not serve as a reinforcer in ACI and F344 rats.[20,21] Unpublished receptor binding studies using these same rat strains indicated that there were no differences in either affinity or number for striatal ^{3}H-GBR 12935 binding to dopamine transporters, ^{3}H-SCH 23390 binding to striatal dopaminergic D_1 receptors or ^{3}H-spiperone binding to striatal dopaminergic D_2 receptors, however. In addition, there were no differences between strains in the affinity of (-)cocaine at ^{3}H-GBR 12935 sites. These results suggest that although the dopamine transporter plays a primary role in determining the reinforcing potency of cocaine in animals for which cocaine serves as a reinforcer, differences in cocaine binding to this site may not account for individual or strain differences in whether or not cocaine will serve as a reinforcer. At least, other experiments designed to assess localized receptor density will be necessary to elucidate the influence of specific dopaminergic neuronal systems on genetic differences in the reinforcing properties of cocaine. These experiments illustrate the importance of multiple research designs, specifically both genetic and pharmacological correlations, to understand the generality of research findings.

Studies of genetic differences in opiate receptor binding illustrate the advantages that one methodology may have over another in elucidating discrete biochemical mechanisms associated with a particular drug effect. In 1975, Baran et al.[22] published the first report of genetic differences in receptor binding for different strains within a species. Specifically, they reported differences among recombinant inbred strains of mice in ^{3}H-naloxone binding to opiate receptors in whole brain homogenates (excluding cerebellums). The results indicated that the CXBK mouse strain, which exhibited the least analgesic response to morphine, had the least number of ^{3}H-naloxone binding sites. Indeed, CXBK mice exhibited 42 percent less receptors than the strain which had the highest number. However, the correlation between opiate receptor number and analgesic response to morphine was positive but not significant across ten strains. More recent research has utilized the development of *in vitro* autoradiography techniques to determine the distribution and relative numbers of multiple opiate receptors in discrete anatomical areas. Moskowitz and colleagues[23,24] have shown that CXBK mice are quite deficient in Mu_1 receptors, particularly in brain regions involved in pain processing. In a recent study, Belknap[25] has also provided autoradiographic evidence that Mu receptor density in the dorsal raphe nucleus is a primary mechanism associated with genetic differences in mouse strains selectively bred for high (HAR) and low (LAR) analgesic response to levorphanol. This localized difference in receptor number was previously entirely masked by crude regional analyses of opiate receptor binding. All of these studies, taken together, illustrate that the selection of the appropriate research methodology can enhance the probability of observing statistically significant relationships between biochemical measurements and correlated behavioral traits, while other research methods tend to mask the same associations. In both series of experiments, autoradiography provided a more sensitive analysis of local differences in receptor number which appear to be significantly related to drug responses. In addition, Belknap[25] has illustrated that the density of at least some opiate receptors in at least in some brain regions is under relatively tight genetic control (heritability value of 32%). This basic information will be important to build upon in future studies of opiate receptor mediation of various behavioral effects.

Biochemical studies of cell membrane bilayer fluidity and the influence of synaptosomal membrane composition on receptor function have provided an informative framework within which to interpret related experimental results. Several of these related pharmacogenetic studies utilized electron paramagnetic resonance methods to test the hypothesis that animals may inherit different synaptosomal membrane traits which mediate effects of ethanol. Goldstein et al.[26] showed that ethanol exhibits greater membrane disordering effects of ethanol on synaptosomal membrane fluidity in Long-Sleep (LS) mice, selectively bred for high sensitivity to hypnotic doses of ethanol, relative to Short-Sleep (SS) mice, bred for low sensitivity to ethanol. Likewise, unpublished data from our laboratory has shown a correlation between brain and blood ethanol concentrations at the time of the loss of the righting reflex (LORR) and innate synaptosomal order parameters (S), determined by electron paramagnetic resonance experiments. Our research indicates approximately 3 percent differences in S values between both rat and mouse strains which were most sensitive to ethanol and those which were least sensitive.

The differences in order parameters found in each of these studies is relatively small. However, these observations are better understood when placed in a framework of previous experimental results concerning biological membranes. First, the S value obtained in electron paramagnetic resonance studies ranges from zero to one, corresponding to the probe floating freely in an organic solvent and to the probe being attached to a slab of granite, respectively. In addition, values between 0.4 and 0.6, approximately, would be associated with a viable organism. Thus, only a very small range of values would encompass the results of any of these experiments. Second, previously published data provide suggestions about the physiological relevance of small changes in membrane fluidity which come to bear on the results of later studies. Trudell et al.[27] showed that the anesthetic effects of alcohol could be reversed by increases in atmospheric pressure. Changes in membrane order parameters associated with pressure in the range of that necessary for partial reversal of anesthesia were approximately 0.5%. Likewise, Chin and Goldstein[28] showed that adding 400 mg/dl ethanol to their membrane preparations decreased synaptosomal order parameters by 0.5%. Third, related evidence concerning lipid-protein interactions indicates that adjacent lipid domains regulate the function of many proteins, including receptors and ion pumps.[29,30,31,32] Furthermore, ethanol has been shown to influence the binding of ligands to their receptors.[33,34] Clearly, the historical perspective concerning the ethanol-membrane and membrane-protein interactions helps to determine that relatively small differences in innate membrane fluidity are likely to be physiologically relevant in influencing neuronal function and subsequent behavioral effects, either in the presence or absence of ethanol.

Finally, several pharmacogenetic studies have illustrated that, as in other areas of scientific endeavor, increasing the number of experimental observations increases the potential generality and statistical significance of experimental results. Recently, several investigators have successfully shown that increasing the number of animal strains in pharmacogenetic experimental designs, both decreases the chances of spurious relationships and facilitates the gain of valuable information from relatively small differences between pairs of strains. In particular, the application of pharmacogenetic methods to the study of ethanol self-administration and ethanol-related phenotypes such as sensitivity to ethanol and ethanol preference has allowed several laboratories to assess the relationship between these phenotypes. This is an especially important application of the power of the pharmacogenetic method because the operant methodology involves a relatively complex task which typically requires relatively long periods of training and testing and that relatively small numbers of subjects be tested simultaneously. By choosing pairs of inbred or selected lines of mice and rats to be used as subjects, each of which represents differences in one or more ethanol-related phenotype, multiple comparisons can be made, thus overcoming the disadvantages of the operant method for pharmacogenetic experiments. The pattern of segregation of phenotypes across studies allows the determination of the relationship between phenotypes.[20,35,36,37,38,39]

Other investigators have also shown the resolving power of using large numbers of rodent strains in determining the relationships between both behavioral and biochemical traits. Many ethanol-related phenotypes were studied in eight inbred rat strains in preparation for the development of the NIH outbred rat strain.[40] These studies allowed the determination of correlations between any pair of traits studied. This experimental approach has also been elegantly applied to studies designed to assess the relationship between various nicotine-induced behavioral phenotypes and several cholinergic nicotinic receptor binding parameters.[41,42,43,44] Utilizing 19 inbred strains of mice in their analysis, these investigators have illustrated that significant differences in receptor number and regional distribution can be consistently observed across strains in *in vitro* receptor binding techniques, even though specific pairwise comparisons are statistically insignificant. Furthermore, using multivariate statistical analyses, these investigators have shown that observed differences in receptor binding are correlated with specific behavioral effects of nicotine. Finally, these studies, like those of Belknap,[25] provide information about the heritability of nicotinic receptor number and regional distribution in inbred mice which will be useful for future analyses of these neuronal systems.

CONCLUSION

In summary, the multidisciplinary nature of pharmacogenetics as a discrete scientific field of endeavor as well as the traditional uses of the scientific methods which are now being applied to pharmacogenetic experiments necessitates careful consideration of many often conflicting theoretical perspectives in the process of interpretation of experimental results. It is thus imperative that results of pharmacogenetic studies are presented and discussed within the context of expectations concerning genetic variance as well as traditional uses and assumptions related to applied methodology. If this approach to publicizing experimental results is not taken, there is a risk that the power of pharmacogenetic models will not generally be recognized by the scientific community as a whole. Most importantly, the expenditures of physical and intellectual time and energy used for these careful analyses will not be matched by the acceptance and incorporation of important results into the appropriate body of scientific literature. Rather, important experimental results may be relegated to the status of scientific obscurity.

REFERENCES

1. Griffiths RR, Bigelow GE and Henningfield JE. Similarities in animal and human drug-taking behavior. In: Mello NK, ed., Advances in Substance Abuse, Vol. 1, JAI Press Inc., 1980; 1-90.

2. Conti-Tronconi BM and Raftery MA. The nicotinic cholinergic receptor: Correlation of molecular structure with functional properties. Ann. Rev. Biochem. 1982; 51: 492-530.

3. Levitan ES, Schofield PR, Burt DR, Rhee LM, Wisden W, Kohler M, Fujita N, Rodriguez HF, Stephenson A, Darlison MG, Barnard EA and Seeburg PH. Structural and functional basis for $GABA_A$ receptor heterogeneity. Nature. 1988; 335: 76-79.

4. Nef P, Mauron A, Stalder R, Alliod C and Balliver M. Structure, linkage, and sequence of the two genes encoding the delta and gamma subunits of the nicotinic acetylcholine receptor. Proc Natl Acad Sci. 1984; 81:7975-7979.

5. Noda M, Furutani Y, Takahashi H, Toyosato M, Tanabe T., Shimizu S, Kikyotami S, Kayano T, Hirose T, Inayamn S and Numa S. Cloning and sequence analysis of calf cDNA and human genomic DNA encoding alpha-subunit precursor of muscle acetylcholine receptor. Nature. 1983; 305:818-823.

6. Schmidt AW and Peroutka SJ. 5-Hydroxytryptamine receptor "families." FASEB. 1989; 3: 2242-2249.

7. Freissmuth M, Casey PJ and Gilman AG. G proteins control diverse pathways of transmembrane signaling. FASEB. 1989; 3: 2125-2131.

8. Belknap JK. Genetic factors in the effects of alcohol: Neurosensitivity, functional tolerance and physical dependence. In: Rigter H and Crabbe JC, ed. Alcohol Tolerance and Dependence. New York, Elsevier/North-Holland Biomedical Press. 1980: 157-180.

9. Crabbe JC and Belknap JK. Pharmacogenetic tools in the study of drug tolerance and dependence. Subst Alc Actions/Misuse. 1980; 1: 385-413.

10. Ritz MC, Lamb RJ, Goldberg SR and Kuhar MJ. Cocaine receptors on dopamine transporters are related to self-administration of cocaine. Science. 1987; 237: 1219-1223.

11. Goeders NE and Smith JE. Reinforcing properties of cocaine in the medial prefrontal cortex: Primary action on presynaptic dopaminergic terminals. Pharmacol. Biochem. Behav. 1986; 25: 191-199.

12. Goeders NE, Dworkin SI and Smith JE. Neuropharmacological assessment of cocaine self-administration into the medical prefrontal cortex. Pharmacol Biochem Behav. 1986; 24: 1429-1440.

13. Goeders N and Smith J. Cortical dopaminergic involvement in cocaine reinforcement. Science. 1983; 221: 773-775.

14. Porrino LJ, Ritz MC, Sharpe LG, Goodman NL, Kuhar MJ and Goldberg SR. Differential effects of pharmacological manipulation of serotonin systems on cocaine and amphetamine self-administration in rats. Life Sci. 1989; 45: 1529-1535.

15. Roberts MCS, Corcoran ME and Fibiger HC. On the role of ascending catecholaminergic systems in intravenous self-administration on cocaine. Pharmacol. Biochem. Behav. 1977; 6: 615-620.

16. Roberts DCS, Koob GF, Klonoff P and Fibiger HC. Extinction and recovery of cocaine self-administration following 6-hydroxydopamine lesions of the nucleus accumbens. Pharmacol. Biochem. Behav. 1980; 12: 781-787.

17. Roberts DCS and Koob GF. Disruption of cocaine self-administration following 6-hydroxydopamine lesions of the ventral tegmental area in rats. Pharmacol. Biochem. Behav. 1982; 17: 901-904.

18. Wise RW. Neural mechanisms of the reinforcing action of cocaine. In: Grabowski J, ed. Cocaine: Pharmacology, effects, and treatment of abuse. NIDA Research Monograph Series, 1984; 50: 15-33.

19. Woolverton WL, Goldberg LI and Ginos JZ. Intravenous self-administration of dopamine receptor agonists by rhesus monkeys. J. Pharmacol. Exp. Ther. 1984; 230: 678-683.

20. George FR and Goldberg SR. Genetic approaches to the analysis of addiction. Trends Pharmacol. Sci. 1989; 10: 78-83.

21. Ritz MC, George Fr, Boja JW and Kuhar MJ. Cocaine binding sites on dopamine transporters: Interaction with other variables mediating reinforcement. NIDA monograph, Proceedings of the 1989 Committee on Problems of Drug Dependence Meeting. 1989; pp. 239-246.

22. Baran A, Shuster L, Eleftheriou BE and Bailey DW. Opiate receptors in mice: Genetic differences. Life Sci. 1975; 17:633-640.

23. Moskowitz A and Goodman RR. Autoradiographic analysis of Mu_1, Mu_2, and delta opioid binding in the central nervous system of C57BL/6By and CXBK (Opioid receptor-deficient) mice. Brain Res. 1985; 360:108-116.

24. Moskowitz A, Terman GW, Carter KR, Morgan MJ and Liebeskind JC. Analgesic, locomotor and lethal effects of morphine in the mouse: Strain comparisons. Brain Res. 1985; 361:46-51.

25. Belknap J. Where are the mu receptors that mediate opioid analgesia?: An autoradiographic study in the HAR and LAR selection lines. Advances Alcohol Subst Abuse, 1990 (in press).

26. Goldstein DB, Chin JH and Lyon RC. Ethanol disordering of spin-labeled mouse brain membranes: Correlation with genetically determined ethanol sensitivity of mice. Proc. Natl. Acad. Sci. 1982; 79: 4231-4233.

27. Trudell JR, Hubbell WL and Cohen EN. Pressure reversal of inhalation

anesthetic-induced disorder in spin-labeled phospholipid vesicles. Biochem. Biophys. Acta. 1973; 291: 328-334.

28. Chin J and Goldstein DB. Effects of low concentrations of ethanol on the fluidity of spin-labeled erythrocytes and brain membranes. Mol. Pharmacol. 1977; 13: 435-441.

29. Craido M, Eibl H, and Barrantes FJ. Effects of lipids on acetylcholine receptor. Essential need of cholesterol for maintenance of agonist-induced state transitions in lipid vesicles. Biochemistry. 1982; 21: 3622-3627.

30. Hasegawa J-I, Loh HH and Lee NM. Lipid requirement for mu opioid receptor binding. J. Neurochem. 1987; 49: 1007-1012.

31. Kimelburg HK. The influence of membrane fluidity on the activity of membrane-bound enzymes. In: Poste G and Nicholson GL, eds. Dynamic aspects of cell surface organization. Elsevier/North Holland Biomedical Press, 1977: 205-293.

32. Yeagle PL. Lipid regulation of cell membrane structure and function. FASEB. 1989; 3: 1833-1842.

33. Khatami S, Hoffman PL, Shibuya T and Salafsky B. Selective effects of ethanol on opiate receptor subtypes in brain. Neuropharm. 1987; 26: 1503-1507.

34. Rapaka RS, Renugopalakrishnan V, Goehl TJ and Collins BJ. Ethanol induced conformational changes of the peptide ligands for the opioid receptors and their relevance to receptor interaction. Life Sci. 1986; 39: 837-842.

35. Elmer GI, Meisch RA and George FR. Differential concentration-response curves for oral ethanol self-administration in C57BL/6J and BALB/cJ mice. Alcohol. 1987; 4: 63-68.

36. Ritz MC, George FR and Meisch RA. Ethanol self-administration in ALKO rats: I. Effects of selection and ethanol concentration. Alcohol. 1989; 6: 227-233.

37. Ritz MC, George FR and Meisch RA. Ethanol self-administration in ALKO rats: II. Effects of selection and fixed-ratio. Alcohol. 1989; 6: 235-239.

38. Suzuki T, George FR and Meisch RA. Differential establishment and maintenance of oral ethanol reinforced behavior in Lewis and Fischer 344 inbred rat strains. J. Pharmacol. Exp. Ther. 1988; 245: 164-170.

39. Waller MB, McBride WJ, Gatto GJ, Lumeng L and Li T-K. Intragastric self-infusion of ethanol by ethanol-preferring and -nonpreferring lines of rats. Science. 1984; 225: 78-80.

40. Spuhler K and Deitrich D. Correlative analysis of ethanol-related phenotypes in rat inbred strains. Alcoholism Clin. Exper. Res. 1984; 8: 480-484.

41. Collins AC and Marks MJ. Progress towards the development of animal models of smoking-related behaviors. Adv Alcohol Subst Abuse. 1990 (in press).

42. Marks MJ, Stitzel J and Collins AC. Genetic influences on nicotinic responses. Pharm. Biochem. Behav. 1989; 33: 667-678.

43. Marks MJ, Romm E, Campbell SM and Collins AC. Variation of nicotinic binding sites among inbred strains. Pharm. Biochem. Behav. 1989; 33: 669-689.

44. Miner LL and Collins AC. Strain comparison of nicotine-induced seizure sensitivity and nicotinic receptors. Pharm Biochem Behav. 1989; 33:469-475.

Genetic Influences in Human Substance Abuse

Roy W. Pickens, PhD
Dace S. Svikis, PhD

SUMMARY. The importance of clinical studies to genetic research on substance abuse is discussed. This paper compares the advantages and limitations of methods employed in clinical studies to those employed in animal studies. It stresses the complementary nature of human and animal studies for improving our understanding of genetic influences in substance abuse. Finally, it reviews findings from adoption and twin studies of substance abuse. Whereas much is known about genetic influences in human alcoholism, relatively little is known about genetic influences in other types of drug abuse. This disparity is directly related to the amount of research that has been conducted in the two areas over the past several years.

Both clinical and animal studies contribute to our understanding of genetic factors in substance abuse. Both types of studies employ controlled methodology and therefore yield equally valid results. However, clinical studies differ from animal studies in several important respects. One obvious difference is in the species involved—clinical studies involve humans rather than animals as research subjects. Clinical studies are also more likely to investigate conditions that arise in the natural environment (e.g., drug abuse), rather than conditions that are created in a research labora-

Roy W. Pickens is associated with the Addiction Research Center, National Institute on Drug Abuse, Baltimore, MD. Dace S. Svikis is associated with the Department of Psychiatry and Behavioral Sciences, The Johns Hopkins University School of Medicine, Baltimore, MD.

The opinions expressed herein are the views of the authors and do not necessarily reflect the official position of the National Institute on Drug Abuse.

Reprint requests may be addressed to Roy W. Pickens, PhD, Addiction Research Center, Building C, Room 392, 4940 Eastern Avenue, Baltimore, MD 21224.

tory (e.g., drug self-administration). Finally, clinical studies are often based on a subject's self-report of symptoms, while animal studies are more likely to involve direct measurement of a behavioral or biological process.

This paper describes clinical methods used in the study of genetic influences in human substance abuse. It compares such methods to those employed in animal studies, and discusses their complementary nature for improving our understanding of genetic influences in substance abuse. Finally, it reviews the current status of research in the area. In the paper, attention is focused on twin and adoption studies as clinical methods for distinguishing genetic and environmental influences. A subsequent paper (Svikis and Pickens, this volume) examines methodological issues and critical assumptions that underlie these methods, and discusses how these issues and assumptions influence validity and generalizability of the results.

CLINICAL VS. ANIMAL RESEARCH

Animal studies appear to have several advantages over clinical studies in genetic research. Their primary advantage lies in providing the investigator with direct control over experimental manipulations. In clinical studies, no direct control is often possible, and investigators must rely on natural events to create the test conditions. In laboratory studies, relatively homogeneous subjects can be used, having been selectively bred or reared under controlled conditions. Humans, on the other hand, are notoriously heterogeneous, both in terms of genetic characteristics as well as past experience. In animal studies, the experimenter can directly measure the effects of the experimental intervention, whereas clinical studies must often rely on subject self-report. Finally, animal studies permit influences to be investigated that cannot be investigated in humans for practical and ethical reasons. Greater public scrutiny is directed toward the use of humans in research. For example, humans cannot be deliberately made drug dependent for the purpose of studying drug dependence, yet such procedures are frequently carried out in animal research.

While animal studies offer several methodological advantages, clinical studies play an equally important role in drug abuse research. Clinical studies deal directly with the issue of human drug abuse, which is the *raison d'être* for public support of drug abuse research. Without human drug abuse, there would be little practical justification for drug abuse research. Research with humans also avoids questions of interspecies generality that arise in animal studies. From a biological perspective, rats, mice, and monkeys differ from humans in many respects, and some of these differences may be important in the etiology of drug abuse. Care must always be taken in generalizing the results of animal studies to humans as different species are involved and drug self-administration occurs under different environmental conditions. Finally, human clinical research allows study of factors that often cannot be practically duplicated with animals under laboratory conditions. For example, psychosocial and cultural factors believed to be important in determining initial onset of human drug abuse are difficult to establish with laboratory animals.

Rather than being antagonistic, animal and clinical studies play complementary roles in the study of genetic factors in substance abuse. Animal studies show what is possible under restricted test conditions, while clinical studies focus more on what actually occurs in the natural environment. Hopefully, findings from the two types of studies will agree. If they do not, then sources of the discrepancy must be found or else questions are raised about validity of the methods. If evidence of genetic factors in substance abuse is found in laboratory animal studies but not in human clinical studies, this would raise questions about the validity of the animal models for study of substance abuse. The reverse would be less troublesome for human clinical studies, as it could be argued that such studies reflect species differences or interactions with variables typically not studied in animal research (i.e., social/cultural influences). Nevertheless, failure to find evidence of genetic influences in human studies after finding such evidence in animal studies may be the result of problems inherent to clinical research, such as problems of heterogeneity and diagnostic classification of human subjects resulting in lack of sensitivity to detect a genetic effect.

CLINICAL RESEARCH METHODOLOGY

Clinical methods often capitalize on naturally occurring events, rather than events arranged in a laboratory, for studying etiological influences in a trait or disorder. Two types of studies for detecting genetic influences are adoption and twin studies. In the adoption study, prevalence of a disorder is determined in two groups of adoptees: offspring of biological parents having the disorder and offspring of biological parents not having the disorder. Since both groups of adoptees are separated from their biological parents early in life and reared by nonaffected adoptive parents, the method largely separates the genetic contributions of the biological parents from the environmental contributions of the adoptive parents. Higher rates of the disorder in adopted-away offspring of biological parents with the disorder than in adopted-away offspring of biological parents without the disorder suggest the presence of genetic factors in the etiology of the disorder.

The second method for separating genetic and environmental influences is the twin study. This method capitalizes on the fact that monozygotic and dizygotic twins differ in terms of number of shared genes. Monozygotic (MZ) twins come from a single fertilized ovum, and therefore both members of a pair share the same genes. However, dizygotic (DZ) twins come from two separately fertilized ova, with both members on the average sharing only about half of their genes. To the extent that both types of twins share equally similar rearing environments, higher concordance for the disorder in MZ than DZ twins suggests the presence of genetic factors in the etiology of the disorder.

Interpretation of results from both adoption and twin studies is influenced by a number of methodological issues and critical assumptions. These will be the subject of the following paper. However, assuming these issues and assumptions are addressed, both methods represent powerful strategies for separating the effects of genes and environment at the human clinical level. Powerful statistical techniques exist that employ data from adoption and twin studies in combination with data on population prevalence of a disorder to estimate the extent to which genetic influences contribute to liability variance.

In addition to adoption and twin methods, other powerful methods are available for identifying the specific risk factors that may be inherited in substance abuse. In the high-risk study design, for example, individuals at high risk are compared to individuals at low risk prior to their entry into the risk period to identify measures that distinguish the two groups. Since children of alcoholics are at higher risk for alcoholism than children of nonalcoholics, differences between the two groups prior to the initiation of regular alcohol use may identify specific risk factors that mediate alcoholic risk. Family pedigree studies also contribute to the identification of genetic influences in substance abuse. Although they cannot distinguish between genetic and environmental effects, family studies are useful genetic research tools. Familial clustering of a disorder is suggestive of genetic influences and allows other methods to then be employed in distinguishing genetic and environmental effects.

MEASURES IN CLINICAL STUDIES

In animal research, evidence of genetic factors in substance abuse is typically suggested by a change in (1) the magnitude of a drug response or (2) the tendency for drug self-administration. An example of the first measure would be breeding mice to show an exaggerated sleeping response to barbiturates. An example of the second measure (i.e., tendency for self-administration) would be testing rats selectively bred for alcohol preference to determine their tendency to self-administer other drugs as well. In clinical studies, similar dependent measures are employed, except the focus of such studies is directed more toward clinical issues. Examples include studies to determine genetic contribution to magnitude of response to antidepressant medication, and testing children of alcoholics to determine if they have an increased tendency to abuse other drugs as well.

One major difference between animal and clinical studies is in measures of drug self-administration. In animal self-administration studies, the dependent measure is typically whether or not a drug will be self-administered. In contrast, clinical studies will often distinguish between multiple types of drug self-administration. This is because a number of social, legal, and other factors are recognized as being important determinants of human drug self-administration. Thus, in clinical studies, distinction may be made between problematic and nonproblematic use, licit and illicit drug use, single and polydrug use, etc. Other distinctions made at the human level are between current or lifetime use, between use that is primary or secondary to a psychiatric condition, between familial or nonfamilial types of drug abusers, etc.

At the human level, not everyone uses drugs, not everyone who uses drugs can be considered a "heavy" drug user, and not everyone who is a heavy user has a clinical disorder. Thus, an important aspect of human clinical studies is distinguishing between types of drug use to determine whether or not an individual has a clinical disorder. Biological markers would be ideal for distinguishing between such individuals. Unfortunately, such markers for substance-use disorders do not as yet exist. Therefore, we must rely on behavioral indicators for diagnostic purposes.

Various systems have been developed over the past several decades for identifying individuals with substance-use disorders. The systems have been increasingly refined as knowledge about the nature of the disorders has evolved. Until recently, the DSM-III system, developed by the American Psychiatric Association, was in widespread use.[1] In the recently announced DSM-III-R system, multiple symptoms are required for the diagnosis of Psychoactive Substance Dependence,[2] including evidence of cognitive, behavioral, or physiological impairment and continued substance use despite adverse drug-related consequences. Specific symptoms include loss of control over use, primacy of substance-use activities, withdrawal symptoms, etc. Over the years, clinical studies have employed a variety of systems for diagnosing substance-use disorders, typically relying on the most recently developed system in common use at the time. This has led to difficulties in generalizing results across studies.

Concomitant with the development of diagnostic criteria has been development of standardized instruments for data collection. Such instruments insure that information is collected in the same manner by different investigators. One example of a standardized instrument for data collection is the Diagnostic Interview Schedule (DIS), which is an epidemiological survey instrument that allows clinical diagnosis by DSM-III and other criteria.[3]

CLINICAL STUDIES OF ALCOHOLISM

A large number of twin and adoption studies have been conducted examining quantity and frequency of alcohol use by members of the general population. Far fewer studies have been conducted of the clinical syndrome of alcoholism. This is because clinical studies are typically large-scale projects and expensive to conduct. Not only must twins or adoptees be located who have substance-use disorders, but information on substance use by their cotwins or by their adoptive and biological parents must be obtained as well. Thus, it is not surprising that there have been relatively few studies in the area. In the brief review to follow, we will summarize the results in general terms, ignoring differences in absolute risk rates that are believed to be due to methodological differences in the studies themselves. The terms "alcoholism" and "drug abuse" will be used generically to refer to a variety of alcohol- and drug-related classification systems that were employed in the various studies.

Most adoption and twin studies of substance-use disorders have involved alcoholism. In the first adoption study of alcoholism, Roe failed to find higher alcoholism rates in the adopted-away offspring of alcoholics than nonalcoholics.[4] However, more recent studies have consistently found that adopted-away sons of alcoholics have higher alcoholism rates than adopted-away sons of nonalcoholics.[5-7] Adoption studies with female adoptees have shown less consistent results. One study found no higher rates of alcoholism in the adopted-away daughters of alcoholics than nonalcoholics,[8] another study found higher alcoholism rates among daughters of alcoholics,[7] and a third study found excessive alcoholism only in a subgroup whose fathers had mild alcoholism with no evidence of criminality.[9]

In twin studies of alcoholism, the results have also been somewhat inconsistent. With males, two of the three previous studies have found higher MZ than DZ concordance rates,[10,11] while the third study found no difference in MZ/DZ concordance rates.[12] With females, only one previous twin study has been conducted and it failed to find higher MZ than DZ concordance rates.[12] However, this was also the same study that failed to find higher MZ than DZ concordance rates in males, and therefore the results are questionable.

In general, both adoption and twin studies of alcoholism show clear evidence of genetic involvement in male alcoholism. In female alcoholism, however, the picture is not as clear, with fewer studies having been conducted and more inconsistent results.

CLINICAL STUDIES OF DRUG ABUSE

Compared to alcoholism, there has been little research on genetic factors in other types of drug abuse.[13] Several factors may account for this, including greater interest in environmental determinants of drug abuse by researchers and funding agencies, lower prevalence rates for drug abuse (compared to alcoholism) in the general population, greater difficulties in working with drug abusers (due to higher rates of criminality and psychopathology), experimental complications arising from prevalence of polydrug use, etc.

Most of the previous clinical studies of genetic factors in drug abuse have focused on use of licit drugs by individuals in the general population (not dependence on illicit drugs by clinical populations). In twin studies of cigarette smoking, several studies have found higher MZ than DZ concordance rates,[14-17] although a study of twins raised apart failed to find MZ and DZ differences.[18] Higher MZ than DZ concordance rates for use of tea, coffee and tranquilizers has also been reported,[17] although the same study failed to find higher MZ than DZ concordance rates for use of sleeping pills. Other twin studies, however, have reported higher MZ than DZ concordance rates for both sleeping pill and tranquilizer use.[17] No other twin study of drug abuse has been reported, except for a case study of a single MZ twin pair which reported one member to be a heavy user of heroin and other illicit drugs, while the other member was drug-free and adamantly opposed to the use of street drugs.[19]

Only one adoption study of drug abuse has been published to date. Cadoret et al. employed DSM-III criteria to identify drug abuse in matched groups of adoptees with and without psychopathology in their first-degree relatives.[20] With data from males and females combined, drug abuse in adoptees was associated with both genetic and environmental factors. For adoptees without antisocial personality, drug abuse was correlated with biological parents having alcohol problems. For adoptees with antisocial personality, drug abuse was correlated with biological parents having antisocial personality. Finally, drug abuse in adoptees was correlated with divorce and psychiatric disturbance in the adoptive family.

CONCLUSIONS

Clearly, more attention must be given to clinical studies of genetic factors in drug abuse. The importance of clinical studies in understanding genetic factors in substance abuse cannot be overemphasized. Not only do such studies advance knowledge in their own right, but they also provide validity for laboratory studies. Hopefully, as the area of genetic factors in drug abuse develops, the results of laboratory and clinical studies will be the same, and the results from the two types of studies will strengthen one another and lead to more rapid advancements in the area.

REFERENCES

1. American Psychiatric Association. *Diagnostic and statistical manual of mental disorders*. Washington, D.C.: American Psychiatric Association, 1981.

2. American Psychiatric Association. *Diagnostic and statistical manual of mental disorders. Third edition – revised*. Washington, D.C.: American Psychiatric Association, 1987.

3. Robins LN, Helzer JE, Croughan J, Ratcliff KS. National Institute of Mental Health diagnostic interview schedule: its history, characteristics, and validity. *Arch. Gen. Psychiatry*. 1981; 38:381-389.

4. Roe A. The adult adjustment of children of alcoholic parents raised in foster homes. *Q. J. Stud. Alcohol*. 1944; 5:378-393.

5. Goodwin DW, Schulsinger F, Hermansen L, et al. Alcohol problems in adoptees raised apart from alcoholic biological parents. *Arch. Gen. Psychiatry*. 1973; 28:238-243.

6. Cloninger CR, Bohman M, Sigvardsson S. Inheritance of alcohol abuse. *Arch. Gen. Psychiatry*. 1981; 38:861-868.

7. Cadoret RJ, Gath A. Inheritance of alcoholism in adoptees. *Br. J. Psychiatry*. 1978; 132:252-258.

8. Goodwin DW, Schulsinger F, Knop J, et al. Alcoholism and depression in adopted-out daughters of alcoholics. *Arch. Gen. Psychiatry*. 1977; 34:751-755.

9. Bohman M, Sigvardsson S, and Cloninger CR. Maternal inheritance of alcohol abuse. *Arch. Gen. Psychiatry*. 1981; 38:965-969.

10. Kaij L. *Alcoholism in twins*. Stockholm: Almqvist and Wiksell, 1960.

11. Hrubec Z, Omenn GS. Evidence of genetic predisposition to alcoholic cirrhosis and psychosis: twin concordances for alcoholism and its biological end points by zygosity among male veterans. *Alcoholism*. 1981; 5:207-215.

12. Gurling HMD, Murray RM, Clifford CA. Investigations into the genetics of alcohol dependence and into its effects on brain function. *Twin research 3: epidemiological and clinical studies*. New York: Alan R. Liss, 1981.

13. Pickens R, Svikis DS. *Biological vulnerability to drug abuse*. NIDA research monograph 89. DHHS publication number (ADM) 88-1590. Washington, DC: US Government Printing Office, 1988.

14. Friberg L, Kaij L, Dencker SJ, Jonsson E. Smoking habits of monozygotic and dizygotic twins. *Br. Med. J.* 1959; 1:1090-1092.

15. Shields J. *Monozygotic twins brought up apart and brought up together.* London: Oxford University Press, 1962.

16. Kaprio J, Koskenvuo M, Sarna S. Cigarette smoking, use of alcohol, and leisure-time physical activity among same-sex adult male twins. *Twin research 3: epidemiological and clinical studies.* New York: Alan R. Liss, 1981:37-46.

17. Pedersen N. Twin similarity for usage of common drugs. *Twin research 3: epidemiological and clinical studies.* New York: Alan R. Liss, 1981:53-59.

18. Kaprio J, Koskenvuo M, Langinvainio H. Finnish twins reared apart. IV: Smoking and drinking habits. A preliminary analysis of the effect of heredity and environment. *Acta Genet. Med. Gemellol. (Roma).* 1984; 33:425-433.

19. Grumet GW. Identical twins discordant for heroin abuse: case report. *J. Clin. Psychiatry.* 1983; 44:457-459.

20. Cadoret RJ, Troughton E, O'Gorman, TW, Heywood E. An adoption study of genetic and environmental factors in drug abuse. *Arch. Gen. Psychiatry.* 1986; 43:1131-1136.

Methodological Issues in Genetic Studies of Human Substance Abuse

Dace S. Svikis, PhD
Roy W. Pickens, PhD

SUMMARY. This paper described a number of critical assumptions and methodological issues that influence the interpretation of data from family, twin and adoption studies of substance abuse. Also, using data from a recent study, it examined the role of one methodological issue (method of zygosity determination) and one critical assumption (representativeness of twins as research subjects) to determine the validity of data in twin studies of substance abuse. The accuracy of the questionnaire methods for zygosity determination in alcoholic twins was similar to that previously reported for nonalcoholic twins. Also, alcoholic twins were found to be representative of both nonalcoholic twins and alcoholics in general.

In the past, most human genetic studies of substance abuse have focused on alcoholism. Increasing attention is now being paid to human genetic studies of other types of substance abuse. Before embarking on such studies, however, it is important to briefly review not only what can be gleaned from human genetic studies of alcoholism (see Pickens and

Dace S. Svikis is associated with the Department of Psychiatry and Behavioral Sciences, The Johns Hopkins University School of Medicine, Baltimore, MD. Roy W. Pickens is associated with the Addiction Research Center, National Institute on Drug Abuse, Baltimore, MD.

Reprint requests may be addressed to Dace S. Svikis, PhD, Alcoholism Treatment Services, D-5-C, Francis Scott Key Medical Center, 4940 Eastern Avenue, Baltimore, MD 21224.

Svikis, this volume), but also to recognize the extent to which such findings are related to the methods employed to obtain them. Relatively small methodological variations across studies, often overlooked by the casual reader, can have a major impact on the studies' results. Such variation can produce differences both in magnitude of effect as well as in showing evidence of a genetic influence. Indeed, this has been the case in the study of genetic factors in alcoholism where inconsistencies in results have been used to question the role of a genetic influence.[1,2] To date, however, little attention has been paid to the study of methodological factors that influence findings from genetic studies of alcoholism or drug abuse.

Because most human genetic studies of alcoholism have employed the twin and adoption methods, it is also important to recognize that both strategies are based on critical assumptions that must be met to permit valid interpretation of their results. If these assumptions are not met, alternative interpretations are possible. While validity of assumptions underlying twin and adoption studies has been examined in studies of nonclinical characteristics (e.g., personality, intelligence, aging)[3,4] and a variety of medical (e.g., cerebral palsy, congenital malformations) and psychiatric (e.g., schizophrenia) disorders,[4,5] their validity has not been examined with alcoholism and other drug abuse. Thus, it is not known if assumptions underlying adoption and twin studies of nonclinical characteristics can be generalized to clinical disorders such as alcoholism and other drug abuse.

There is reason to believe that such findings may not be generalizable. One major reason for this is the social stigma attached to alcoholism and drug abuse. This stigma may lead to misclassification of research subjects which will increase the difficulty of finding a genetic effect. In twin research, for example, zygosity is often based on self-report of pair similarity. While this method is highly accurate in characterizing twins when traits such as personality and intelligence are studied, when a stigmatized disorder such as alcoholism and other drug abuse is involved, the nonaffected member of a discordant pair may be reluctant to report him/herself as being similar to his/her affected cotwin.[6] Thus, discordant twins may be incorrectly classified as DZ solely on the basis of their discordance for the disorder. The same may also be true in adoption studies, where biological mothers may be unwilling to divulge alcoholism and other drug use/abuse in the biological father. Hence, some adoptees with alcoholic biological fathers may incorrectly be classified as controls, because accurate information on the father's alcohol/drug use was not provided.

Certain methodological issues are common to all types of human genetic studies of substance abuse (see Table 1). A comprehensive review of such issues has recently been published.[6] Thus, they are described below merely to illustrate the nature and scope of such factors in genetic studies of substance abuse. Each issue should be considered in a study's design as it may exert an important influence on the results that are obtained. For example, a study must have an adequate sample size to generate sufficient power for data analysis. Subjects should be recruited in a manner to eliminate bias as much as possible and be representative of the population to which the results will be generalized. Objective and valid criteria for diagnosis of the disorder and standardized methods of data collection should be employed. Subjects should have passed the age of risk for the disorder before they are included in the sample. Age, gender, psychiatric comorbidity and drug use by subjects should also be considered in both data collection and analysis.

Other methodological issues are specific to twin studies and adoption studies. In twin studies, they include accuracy of method for zygosity determination, representativeness of twins to nontwins, the assumption of equal similarity in rearing environments for MZ and DZ twins, and random (parental) mating. For adoption studies, they include informant bias, controlling for prenatal and early environmental influences, representativeness of adoptees to nonadoptees, controlling for selective placement of

Table 1

General Methodological Issues
in Human Studies of Substance Abuse

- Adequate Sample Size
- Recruitment Bias
- Diagnostic Criteria
- Method of Data Collection
- Age of Risk
- Gender Differences
- Psychiatric Comorbidity
- Drug Specificity
- Drug Availability

adoptees in adoptive homes, and the assumption of random parental mating.

RECENT RESEARCH

We recently examined several methodological issues and critical assumptions in a twin study of substance abuse. The present study reports the accuracy of various methods for determining zygosity in alcoholic twins, and the validity of the assumption that alcoholic twins are representative of twins in general and alcoholics in particular. Accurate zygosity assessment (i.e., determining if twins are MZ or DZ) is essential to the twin method. For genetically-determined traits, misclassification of MZ twins as DZ and vice versa will decrease the magnitude of the genetic effect by producing lower correlations for MZ twins and higher correlations for DZ twins. A critical assumption underlying all twin research is that twins are representative of nontwins. If this assumption is valid, then data obtained from twin studies can be expected to generalize to the population at large. If the assumption is invalid, then the utility of data obtained from twins remains questionable.

The twins employed in the study were selected from admissions to 16 alcohol and drug treatment or followup programs in the state of Minnesota. The twins and their cotwins were initially administered a written questionnaire and later personally interviewed to obtain information about alcohol and drug use, and other psychiatric disorders. Whenever possible, a 20 ml blood sample was obtained from both members of a twin pair for zygosity determination.

Zygosity Determination. Several methods have been employed to ascertain zygosity, including twin self-report of their own belief concerning zygosity, physical appearance comparisons, questionnaire items about twin similarity (e.g., "Are you and your twin as alike as two peas in a pod?"), and serological analysis. While the most accurate method is serological analysis (in a U.S. sample, 99.9% accurate when 18 blood factors are examined),[7] it is both time consuming and expensive to collect blood samples from both members of all twins participating in a study. Also, with the increasing rates of HIV infection among IV drug users, special precautions must be taken in obtaining and analyzing blood samples for zygosity determination. The accuracy of the other less intrusive methods varies from 60% for twin self-report of belief about zygosity[8,9] to 83-98% for questionnaire items on twin similarity.[10-13]

The study is based on data from the first 108 twin pairs returning the questionnaire and also providing a 20 ml blood sample. Accuracy of two methods for determining zygosity was examined. The first method involved a questionnaire item that simply asked about the type of twin they were (i.e., if they were identical or fraternal). The second involved two questionnaire items that asked about their similarity as children.

In the first method, self-report of type of twin, zygosity was determined by proband/cotwin agreement. If both indicated "identical," the pair was labelled MZ; if both indicated fraternal, the pair was labelled DZ. If either twin reported "don't know" or if they disagreed on zygosity, status the twins were labelled "unclassifiable."

The second method, classifying twins as MZ or DZ based on report of childhood similarity, compared twins on the basis of their responses to the following two items: (a) as children, were you as alike as two peas in a pod, and (b) as children, did even family members have difficulty telling you apart (see Table 2). For each member of a twin pair, responses to each item were quantified (0-2) and then summed to yield a composite similarity score using the same standardized methods employed in previous twin studies: a twin pair was classified MZ if both members of a pair obtained 3 or more total points and DZ if both members obtained 2 or less total

Table 2

Questionnaire Items on Childhood Similarity
Administered Separately to Individual Members of a Twin Pair

1) When you were children, were you and your twin as alike as "two peas in a pod", or were you no more alike than ordinary brothers or sisters? (check one)

_____ Like "two peas"	(2 points)
_____ Ordinary likeness	(1 point)
_____ Quite unlike	(0 points)

2) When you were children, were you and your twin similar enough in appearance so that people had difficulty telling you apart? (check one)

_____ Never had difficulty telling us apart	(0 points)
_____ Sometimes had difficulty telling us apart	(1 point)
_____ Even family members had difficulty telling us apart	(2 points)

points. If one member of a pair obtained 3 or more total points while the other obtained 2 or less total points, the pair was considered unclassifiable by this method.

The accuracy of the two methods for zygosity determination was compared to accuracy based on analyses of 12 serological factors: four red blood cell antigens, four serum proteins, and four red blood cell enzymes. Twins were considered MZ if all blood factors were identical, and DZ if they differed in one or more of these factors. In a study of individuals with similar sociodemographic background, Lykken reported that the probability of this method incorrectly classifying a DZ as a MZ was less than .001.[7]

The results are shown in Table 3. Accuracy rates were calculated separately using proband data only, cotwin data only, and data from both members of a twin pair. For the total sample (categorizing unclassifiable cases as incorrect responses), the accuracy of self-reported zygosity ranged from 72% (when data from both members of a twin pair were considered) to 78% (when data from only the proband were employed) to 81% (when data from only the cotwin were employed), rates similar to those found in twin studies of nonclinical traits. The accuracy of the twin similarity questions ranged from 87% (when data from both members of a twin pair were considered) to 91% (when data from the proband only were considered) to 93% (when data from the cotwin only were taken into account). These rates were also similar to those previously reported in nonclinical studies of twins. The accuracy rate for twin similarity questions was significantly higher than that for self-report ($p < .01$). However, both methods yielded accuracy rates significantly lower than that for serological analyses ($p < .001$).

Thus, the accuracy rates of both methods of zygosity determination in alcoholic twins fell within the range of those reported previously for nonalcoholic twins. While zygosity determination based on pair similarity as children was more accurate than that of self-report, both methods were less accurate than zygosity determination based on serological analysis. While the latter has greater accuracy, such methods are expensive and cannot always be obtained. Using questionnaire items concerning pair similarity as children provide an attractive alternative for zygosity determination, with a misclassification rate of only 7-13%. The present findings extend the generality of these methods to alcoholic twins, and suggest that such methods can be used confidently in future twin studies of alcoholism if serological analysis is not practical.

Alcoholic Twin Representativeness. The representativeness of twins has

Table 3

Accuracy of Different Methods
for Zygosity Determination

	SOURCE OF INFORMATION		
	Proband Only	Cotwin Only	Both
Self-Reported Zygosity	78%	81%	72%
Childhood Similarity	91%	93%	87%

(N=108 pairs)

been studied extensively in nonclinical samples of twins. Twins have been found to differ from singletons on a variety of characteristics (e.g., cognitive abilities). These differences, however, have not been shown to influence significantly the generalizability of twin data to the general population. For example, while twins have a lower mean IQ (96) than has been reported in the general population (100), the variance for the two groups is approximately equal. Thus the range and variability of intellectual abilities among twins is not restricted, indicating that data from twins and singletons can be statistically compared.[14]

While the assumption has been studied intensively in twins from the general population, little is known about the representativeness of alcoholic twins. Two important issues must be addressed in testing the validity of this assumption. First, to what extent are substance abusing twins representative of twins in general? Second, to what extent are twins with substance abuse problems representative of substance abusers in general? The present study tested the validity of these assumptions in a clinical sample of alcoholic twins.

To establish the validity of the first assumption, it is important to show that twins with substance abuse disorders do not differ significantly from twins without the disorder. That is, twinning and the disorder of interest must be shown to be independent, such that being a twin does not influence one's risk for developing the disorder. This assumption has been studied in twins with different psychiatric conditions, and while its validity has been supported for certain disorders (e.g., adult-onset schizophrenia),[15] it has not been substantiated for other disorders (e.g., infantile autism). For the latter, rates of infantile autism are significantly higher in twins than in nontwins,[5,16] suggesting data from autistic twins may not generalize to the population at large.

To examine the representativeness of alcoholic twins to twins in general, the present study compared: (1) twinning rates in a treatment-based sample of alcoholics with twinning rates in the general population and (2) zygosity rates (MZ/same-sex DZ ratios) in alcoholic twins and twins in the general population.

First, the rate of twinning in a substance abuse treatment sample was calculated by comparing the number of twins ascertained at each of the 16 treatment facilities participating in the study to the total number of individuals screened at each program. Data were collected from February, 1985 to June, 1986 and the results are summarized in Table 4. During this time, a total of 337 twins were ascertained from 20,562 patients screened for the study. While twinning rates varied considerably across sites (rang-

Table 4

Twinning Rate in Various Treatment Programs

Treatment Center	Number of Twins	Number Screened	Rate of Twinning
Abbott-NW Hospital	24	921	2.6%
Anoka State Hospital	10	817	1.2%
Brainerd State Hospital	10	810	1.2%
CATOR (Adult)	48	2,955	1.6%
CATOR (Adolescent)	7	795	0.9%
Fergus Falls State Hospital	28	1,898	1.5%
Hazelden (Center City)	41	2,407	1.7%
Hennepin A.I.D.	31	1,444	2.1%
Hennepin Detox	26	3,300	0.7%
Mounds Park Hospital	13	862	1.5%
Hazelden Pioneer House	15	930	1.6%
St. John's Hospital	30	1,095	2.7%
St. Mary's Hospital	21	1,269	1.6%
St. Paul Ramsey Hospital	12	187	6.4%
St. Peter State Hospital	16	774	2.1%
Univ. of Minnesota Hospitals	5	98	5.1%
TOTAL:	**337**	**20,562**	**1.6%**

ing from 0.7% in one program to 6.4% in another), the overall twinning rate was 1.6% which did not differ significantly from the twinning rate of 1.2% reported in the general population.[5]

Second, the zygosity rates for same-sex twin probands ascertained in the study were compared to zygosity rates reported in the general population. For twins admitted for substance abuse treatment, zygosity rates were 47% and 53%, respectively, for MZ and same-sex DZ twins. These rates were within the general population rates of 46-51% for MZ and 49-54% for same-sex DZ twins.[14]

To examine the validity of the second assumption, that alcoholic twins are representative of alcoholics in general, it is important to compare alcoholism characteristics in twins and general patients. If the two samples are similar for such variables, this would suggest that alcoholic twins are representative of alcoholics in general.

The selection of variables appropriate for twin versus general patient population comparisons was difficult because the range of many variables was restricted due to sample characteristics (e.g., in each case, twin proband alcoholism was severe enough to warrant treatment). To minimize this potential bias, characteristics largely unrelated to treatment admission (e.g., demographics, type of substance abuse) were selected for study. Also, general patient population data were available only for patients admitted to the Hazelden drug treatment program, therefore, only twins ascertained at this program site were included in these comparisons.

Hazelden general patient data were available only for 1976 (N = 1,627 patients)[17] and 1985 (N = 1,626 patients).[18] The average of these two years was compared to the characteristics of the Hazelden twins, who were recruited between 1976 and 1986. The variables examined included gender, age at admission, marital status, educational level, and type of substance abuse (e.g., alcohol only, drugs only or alcohol and drugs). A summary of these characteristics for Hazelden patients and Hazelden twins is shown in Table 5. Except for age at admission to treatment, no statistically significant differences were found between the Hazelden general patient population and Hazelden twin probands for these characteristics.

These data generally support the validity of the assumption that alcoholic twins are representative of twins in general and alcoholics in particular. Thus, the data from twin studies of alcoholism should generalize to the general alcoholic population. The findings also support the use of the twin paradigm in studies of genetic factors in alcoholism. These data sug-

Table 5

Demographic Characteristics of Hazelden Patients

Variable	Treatment Population* (N=3253)	Twin Sample (N=75)	p values
Sex			
Males	70%	65%	N.S.
Females	30%	35%	
Admission Age			
Under 26	14%	20%	<.05
26-55	73%	76%	
Over 55	14%	4%	

TABLE 5 (continued)

Variable	Treatment Population* (N=3253)	Twin Sample (N=75)	p values
Marital Status			
Married	50%	49%	N.S.
Single	27%	28%	
Sep./Divorced	20%	20%	
Widowed	3%	3%	
Education Level			
< High School	10%	11%	N.S.
H.S. Graduate	25%	21%	
Some College	24%	33%	
College Graduate	40%	35%	
Substance Abuse			
Alcohol Only	44%	55%	N.S.
Drugs Only	4%	4%	
Both	52%	41%	

* mean of 1976 and 1985 admissions

gest that the assumption of representativeness may also be valid in twin studies of other types of substance use.

CONCLUSIONS

Research results are inextricably related to the methods used to obtain them. Interpretation of findings is also related to the critical assumptions on which the research methods are based. Research in the area of genetic factors in human substance abuse is still in its infancy, and therefore inconsistencies in findings are common. To a significant extent, these inconsistencies are related to different methodologies that have been employed in the relatively few studies that have been conducted in the area. Hopefully, as the number of human genetic studies in the substance abuse area increases, systematic replication and attention to critical assumptions will lead to greater consistency of results and more confidence in interpretation of the findings. Until this occurs, results should be interpreted with caution, and care must be taken to avoid overinterpreting and overgeneralizing the results.

REFERENCES

1. Searles JS. The role of genetics in the pathogenesis of alcoholism. J. Abnorm. Psychol. 1988; 97:153-167.
2. Murray RM, Clifford C, Gurling HM. Twin and adoption studies: How good is the evidence for a genetic role? Recent Dev. Alcohol. 1983; 1:25-48.
3. Plomin R, DeFries JC, McClearn GE. Behavioral genetics: a primer. San Francisco: WH Freeman & Company, 1980.
4. Thompson JS, Thompson MW. Genetics in medicine. Philadelphia: WB Saunders Company, 1980.
5. Gottesman II, Shields J. Schizophrenia: the epigenetic puzzle. Cambridge, MA: Cambridge University Press, 1982.
6. Svikis DS, Pickens RW. Methodological issues in family, adoption and twin research. In: Pickens R. and Svikis D. (eds.), Biological vulnerability to drug abuse. NIDA Res Monograph #89. Washington, DC: US Government Printing Office, 1988: pp. 120-133.
7. Lykken DT. The diagnosis of zygosity in twins. Behav. Genet. 1978; 8:437-473.
8. Carter-Saltzman L, Scarr S. MZ or DZ? Only your blood grouping laboratory knows for sure. Behav. Genet. 1977; 7:273-280.
9. Nichols RC, Bilbro WC. The diagnosis of twin zygosity. Acta Genet. Med. Gemellol. (Roma). 1966; 16:265-275.

10. Segal NL. Zygosity testing: Laboratory and the investigator's judgment. Acta Genet. Med. Gemellol. (Roma). 1984; 33:515-521.
11. Cederlof R, Friberg L, Jonsson E, Kaij L. Studies on similarity of diagnosis with the aid of mailed questionnaires. Acta Genet. Med. Gemellol. (Roma). 1961; 11:338-362.
12. Cohen DJ, Dibble E, Grawe JM, Pollin W. Separating identical from fraternal twins. Arch. Gen. Psychiatry. 1973; 29:465-469.
13. Sarna S, Kaprio J, Sistonen P, Koskenvuo M. Diagnosis of twin zygosity by mailed questionnaire. Hum. Hered. 1978; 28:241-254.
14. Fuller JL, Thompson WR. Foundations of behavior genetics. St. Louis: CV Mosby, 1978.
15. Reveley A. Phenomenology, environmental risk, and genetics: twin studies of schizophrenia. Paper presented at American Psychopathological Association Meeting, New York, 1990.
16. Kallmann FH, Roth B. Genetic aspects of preadolescent schizophrenia. Am. J. Psychiatry. 1956; 112:599-606.
17. Patton MQ. The outcomes of treatment: a study of patients admitted to Hazelden in 1976. Minneapolis: Hazelden Press, 1979.
18. Novalany C. Hazelden primary 1985 patient profile. Minneapolis: Hazelden Press, 1986.

The Use of Nonneuronal Cells as an *In Vitro* Model System for Studying the Genetic Component of Cellular Response to Opiates and Other Drugs of Abuse

John J. Madden, PhD
Arthur Falek, PhD

SUMMARY. Nonneuronal cells, such as the human T lymphocyte, react directly with opiates *in vitro* causing significant alterations in the metabolism of these cells. Morphine and cocaine, for example, can modulate the repair of DNA damage caused by ultraviolet light (UVC) – morphine in the negative direction and cocaine in the positive. The mechanism by which these drugs cause these metabolic changes is not yet known, but a simple receptor mechanism such as is found in the central nervous system (CNS) can not be demonstrated. Binding studies using lymphocyte membrane preparations or whole cells do not support the premise that T lymphocytes have opiate binding sites with specificities comparable to those identified in the CNS – the mu, delta and kappa receptors. Even without knowing the mechanism for the opiate-induced metabolic changes, the alterations can be used as the basis for a test of the genetics of opiate metabolism. If the interindividual variation in the opiate-induced repair response is greater than the intraindividual variation as assessed by repeated measures on the same subject, it may be possi-

---

John J. Madden and Arthur Falek are affiliated with the Department of Psychiatry, Emory University, Atlanta, GA 30322 and with the Human and Behavioral Genetics Laboratory, Georgia Mental Health Institute, 1256 Briarcliff Rd., N.E., Atlanta, GA 30306.

Reprint requests may be addressed to Dr. John J. Madden, at the above address.

This project was supported by NIDA Grants DA-05002 and DA-01451.

ble to utilize this assay in the classic sorts of family or twin studies to determine the genetic component of the response to opiates.

While the contribution of genetics to human alcoholism has been accessible to study through the use of biochemical, physiologic and behavioral models, our understanding of the genetic influences underlying human drug abuse has been limited almost entirely to behavioral and epidemiologic studies. On the one hand, alcoholism can be studied in available human tissues like the liver and peripheral blood, and this has led to a variety of efforts to link biochemical responses to genetic factors. On the other hand, the deficit in biochemical and pharmacological drug abuse studies is attributable to the lack of tissue from the central nervous system (CNS) where there are specific receptors for these drugs. Studies on human brain tissue have generally been limited to difficult-to-obtain, autopsied material,[1] making the study of familial and genetic relationships all but impossible. In such genetic diseases as Huntington's Disease, where brain banks have been set up to collect material to study the genetic and biochemical basis of the disorder, the number of brains collected in the entire United States in a given year is on the order of a dozen or so. To collect even these few requires constant solicitation through the relevant lay society, the Huntington's Disease Society of America. Even if a significantly larger number of brains could be obtained each year, collection of the genetically relevant brains, e.g., siblings, twins, parents, etc., would still be extremely limited. Therefore, if the genetic component of opiate abuse is to be studied in humans, other model tissues must be used because of the difficulty of CNS tissue collection.

Fortunately while nervous system tissue is the traditional site of opiate activity, recent research has spotlighted the immune systems as another focus of opiate action. The human T lymphocyte, for example, reacts to the presence of opiates by alteration of its surface antigens including CD4, CD8 and particularly CD2, the sheep erythrocyte pan T receptor involved in cell division. Other opiate effects have been reported for B cells, monocytes, polymorphonuclear leukocytes, platelets, erythrocytes and even compliment as reviewed in Shibaga and Goldstein,[2] and Madden and Donahoe.[3] While it is clear that it is the opiate that is directly involved *in vitro* in causing the antigenic modulation, the effects on the immune system *in vivo* may in some cases be mediated through opiate receptor systems of the CNS.[4] In fact, mechanistic studies are currently underway in many laboratories to understand the etiology of both *in vivo* and *in vitro* immunomodulation to determine their commonalities and dissimilarities. The potential mediation of the CNS notwithstanding, the directly immunomodulatory effects of opiates and cocaine can be studied *in vitro* and have been shown to be physiologically significant.[2] Therefore this suggests that peripheral blood cells can potentially serve as readily available models to study the genetic control of response to drugs of abuse.

THE MECHANISM OF ACTION OF OPIATES ON T LYMPHOCYTES

While the purification and sequence analyses of the CNS opiate receptors have proven more difficult than first expected, the existence of at least three pharmacologically distinct opiate receptors (mu, delta and kappa) in the CNS is well established. The natural ligands for these receptors are known (B-endorphin, the enkephalins and dynorphin respectively) and the consequences for the binding of these ligands to the receptors in terms of signal transduction and secondary messenger production are well studied. Thus, when the initial reports on the effects of opiates on the immune systems were first published, it was generally assumed, and even expressed, that the pharmacologic mechanism must be the same for both systems because of the expected conservancy of nature. Many of the early experiments, as for example the now classic study of Wybran et al.[5,16] on the effects of morphine and met^5-enkephalin on active E rosetting, and their reversal by naloxone, provided confidence that the opiate was acting through a receptor mechanism comparable to that found in the CNS. Mehrishi and Mills[6] added to this confidence in the existence of lymphocyte receptors by reporting that lymphocytes had a specific binding site for naloxone in the nanomolar concentration range. Madden et al.[7] then reported a saturable naloxone binding site on the T lymphocyte with a K_D of approx. 50 nM. The naloxone was displaceable from this site by a variety of opiate ligands including morphine and several enkephalin derivatives suggesting that indeed there were mu- and delta-like opiate binding sites on the human T lymphocyte. Farrar et al.[8] confirmed these findings, while Mendelsohn et al.[9] did not find saturable naloxone binding possibly because of a high degree of contaminating monocytes. There have now been a number of reports supporting the presence of mu, delta, kappa and even sigma receptors on various T lymphocyte preparations,[3] although much of the data are either incomplete or not fully reported, particularly in terms of showing the actual binding curves or derived curves, such as the Scatchard or Hill plots for calculating the binding parameters.[3]

In our recent experiments attempting to confirm the presence of mu or delta receptors on T cells, we have been unable to demonstrate saturable, specific binding using a variety of mu and delta opiate ligands at physiologically reasonable concentrations—with the exception of (−)-naloxone. Morphine for example will displace naloxone(^{3}H) from a sonicated-cell membrane preparation, but with an IC_{50} of approx. 500nM. This is substantially higher than the K_D of morphine for the CNS mu receptor (1-2 nM) and is quite high compared to the maximal blood concentration after a standard dose capable of producing analgesia. Binding constants or biological responses significantly above the maximum physiologic blood values have little biological relevance and for purposes of genetic research can be ignored. Other mu-specific ligands such as morphiceptin were almost totally ineffective in displacing naloxone. Since displacement of naloxone, a traditional property of CNS mu receptors, occurs only at the physiologically unreasonable concentrations or not at all, it must be concluded that, in the absence of specific binding data from Carr et al.,[10] a traditional mu binding site does not exist on T lymphocytes.

A delta/enkephalin site has been reported by two groups;[11,12] but data have only been fully presented by Zozula et al.[11] Our attempts to displace naloxone(^{3}H) with D-ala^2, D-leu^5-enkephalin (DADLE) or naltrindone (NTI), a specific delta antagonist, were not successful. When DADLE(^{3}H) was used as the labeled ligand, neither DADLE nor NTI caused saturable, specific displacement. Variations in the type of assay (filter or centrifugation) and the assay conditions (temperature and media) did not noticeably improve the results. Further elaboration on the assay methodology are needed from those who have published positive results in order to clear up this apparent discrepancy. Kappa receptor ligands, including bremazocine and U50,488 were also ineffective in displacing naloxone over a very wide range of concentration (10^{-9} to 10^{-4}M), eliminating the possibility that the naloxone was bound to a kappa receptor.

Until well described protocols are published, it must be concluded that the case for mu, delta and kappa opiate binding sites on human T lymphocytes has not been conclusively demonstrated. Until opiate binding studies are published which fully document a case for opiate receptors on human T lymphocytes, other mechanisms must be invoked to explain the potent and dose-dependent drug effects noted on metabolism and immune function.

METABOLIC EFFECTS OF OPIATES ON T LYMPHOCYTES

Beyond the immunologically-defined cell surface effects of opiates on immune system cells, two other assay systems have been employed successfully to detect internal changes caused by opiate action on lymphocytes—DNA repair and mitogen-induced blastogenesis. DNA repair, or more accurately the repair of mutagenic damage to DNA, was first investigated *in vivo* after it was reported that lymphocytes from street heroin addicts carried a higher level of chromosome damage[13] and sister chromatid exchange frequency (SCE)[14] than did cells from non-addicts. When lymphocytes from addicts were then tested for their ability to repair either damage from either ultraviolet light (254nm, UVC) or 8-methoxy psoralen and near ultraviolet light (UVA), the treated cells showed a significantly diminished capacity for repair.[15] This reduction in repair capacity as well as the addict milieu (smoking, poor nutrition and generally poor health) is sufficient to account for the increase in chromosome damage seen in the addicts. These experiments were then extended to an *in vitro* model to determine which types of opiate ligands, and at what concentrations, were effective in mimicking the repair depression seen in street addicts exposed to opiates *in vivo*.

In the *in vitro* opiate treatment repair experiments, the lymphocytes from a pheresis procedure were purified using discontinuous sedimentation on Ficoll; washed exhaustively to remove contaminating Ficoll and endogenous opioids; and used fresh or stored frozen at -120°C before use. Freezing did not alter either repair capacity nor antigen expression (data not shown). The cells were then incubated in Hank's Balanced Salt Solution (HBSS) at 4°C for periods of time from 1 to 18 hr with varying concentrations of opiate. The cells were harvested by centrifugation, washed in fresh buffer containing opiate, counted and diluted to 1×10^7 cells per ml. An aliquot of cells (0.5 ml) were irradiated with 0 to 40 J/m^2 (primarily 20 J/m^2 unless noted), tritiated thymidine added and the mixture incubated for 2 hr. Incorporation of the radioactivity into the repaired areas was quantitated by autoradiography and counting of the number of grains found in each of 100 cells.

Dramatic alterations in repair capacity were found for a number of drugs—morphine, cocaine, and levorphanol—in both the negative *and* positive direction. Morphine incubation, for either 1 hr or 18 hr, profoundly depressed UV-induced repair with a K_D somewhere near 2×10^{-10}M (Figure 1). If T lymphocytes (the predominant cell in the assay > 90%) had a mu receptor similar to that found in the CNS, this assay result would be in close agreement with the binding results reported for the CNS receptor. Unfortunately, no really complete data has yet been presented to demonstrate the presence of a similar binding site on the T lymphocyte for morphine making the mechanism for this physiologically significant effect obscure.

While morphine had a profound negative effect on the repair capacity of

FIGURE 1. Inhibition of UV induced DNA repair by morphine. Lymphocytes were treated with morphine for 1 hr at 4°C immediately prior to UV treatment and the addition of the tritiated thymidine. The points shown represent the mean grain count and s.e.m. for 100 cells. Using the Student t test, those points marked with a + had $p < 0.05$ and those with a * had a $p < 0.01$, when compared with the cells incubated without drug. Where applicable, drug was present thoughout the entire DNA repair assay.

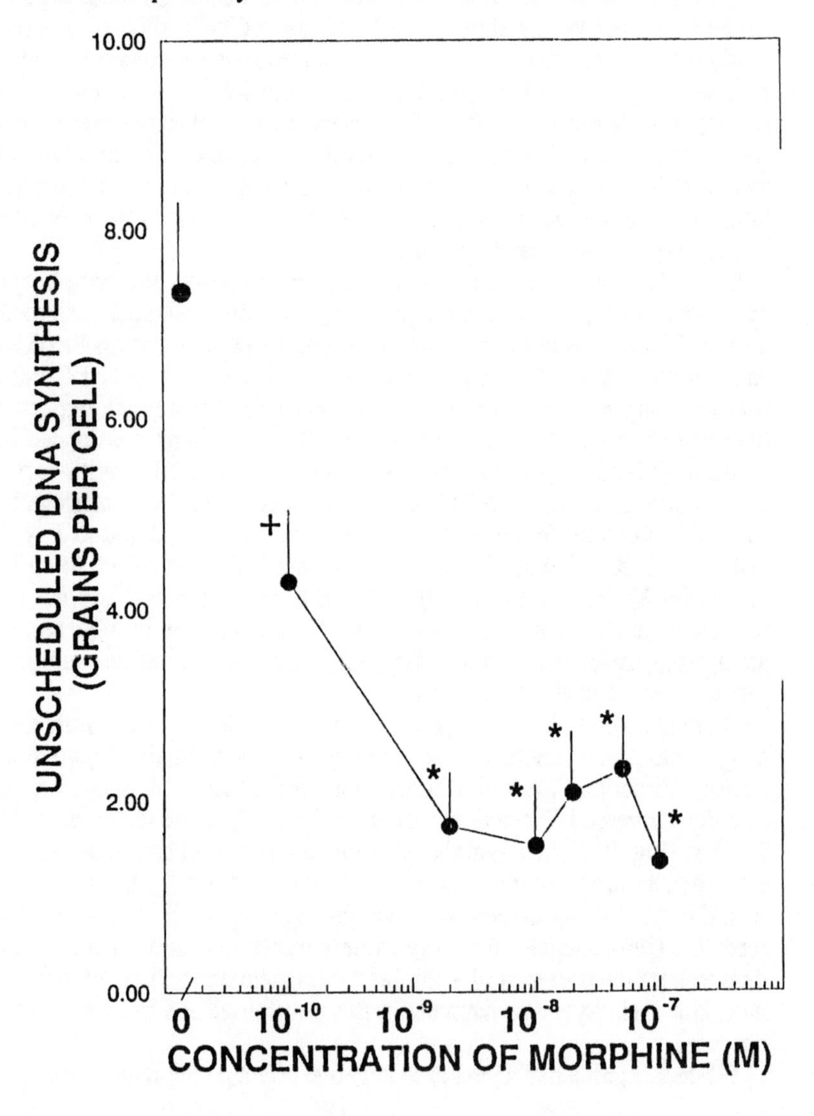

the lymphocyte, cocaine remarkably had the exact opposite effect on repair—instead of decreasing repair, it *increased* it. This was not a totally unexpected result, because a survey of repair capacity of cocaine-abusing, heroin addicts yielded a mean ± standard deviation) of 6.2 ± 4.9 grains/cell compared to a control (nonaddict) population capacity of 2.7 ± 1.5 grains/cell for a standard UV challenge of 20 J/m^2. In the *in vitro* results, doses of cocaine between 10^{-8} to 10^{-7}M yielded a maximum increase over untreated cell capacity of 2-3 fold. In a typical experiment a dose of 10^{-7}M cocaine produced a value of 13.8 ± 7.8 grains/cell; 10^{-8}M yielded 12.0 ± 4.5; 10^{-9}M 8.9 ± 3.2; 10^{-10}M 7.2 ± 3.1; 10^{-11}M 6.2 ± 3.4; while the untreated cells had 6.5 ± 4.2 grains/cell. The increases at 10^{-7} and 10^{-8}M were significant at a p level < 0.01 using the Student t test, while at 10^{-9}M the increase was significant at the 0.05 level. This ability of cocaine to cause such a dramatic increase in apparent repair capacity is currently unique among substances known to affect repair, and its biological significance must be determined. Interestingly, as the concentration of cocaine is raised from 10^{-6} to 10^{-5}M, the cells lost viability as judged by trypan blue exclusion and repair fell to essentially zero in some assays (1.5 ± 3.1 and 0.9 ± 2.2 grains/cell respectively). Several other drugs tested also produced deleterious effects on the lymphocytes at concentration above those that are physiologically reasonable for that drug. These non-specific depressions in lymphocyte function which occur at physiologically unreasonable drug concentration should not be confused with the immune system modulations and metabolic alterations which occur at physiologically attainable levels of specific drugs. At outrageous concentrations virtually everything seems to damage the immune system *in vitro*; but the biological significance of such damage is dubious at best. Therefore the significance of the morphine and cocaine effects on repair in the lymphocyte is that the effects are dose dependent in a concentration range that is physiologically reasonable for both dugs. The physiological significance of the increase in repair caused by cocaine is not clear because it cannot be determined from UDS alone whether the repair is error-free or not. For this reason, cocaine would make an interesting test drug in a mutation rate assay using lymphocytes or lymphoid-derived cell lines.

Experiments with levorphanol further complicate the pattern of DNA repair modulation by drugs of abuse. After a 1 hr incubation of the lymphocytes with levorphanol, repair is significantly depressed, as with morphine, in the range from 10^{-12} to 10^{-6}M. However, after an 18 hr incubation concentration between 10^{-8} and 10^{-5}M appear to be stimulative like cocaine. Further work is obviously needed on incubation time and media conditions to understand the molecular basis for these repair modulations.

While it may appear from the foregoing that all drugs and opiates modulate lymphocyte DNA repair, several significant drugs do not. Naloxone, the opiate antagonist, has no repair modulating capacity over a broad range of concentrations (10^{-11} to 10^{-5}M). Delta-specific opiate ligands, including leu^5-enkephalin, DADLE and leu^5-enkephalinamide, were ineffective in modulating repair at concentrations between 10^{-11} and 10^{-8}M. Various combinations of drugs, such as morphine or cocaine in combination with micromolar concentrations of naloxone, proved to be unexpectedly toxic to the cells making evaluation of repair biologically insignificant. Therefore, there are significant effects of drugs of abuse on the metabolic life of T lymphocytes. However, it is not yet apparent from the structure of the drug and its known biological potency in the CNS, which drugs will have what effects on the lymphocyte and what range of concentrations will be effective. Other compounds must be tested before this pattern becomes apparent.

In trying to discern the mechanism(s) by which the morphine and cocaine modulate repair in the T lymphocyte, two types of experiments have been useful in clarifying possibilities. First, the rate and extent of tritiated thymidine uptake was measured in control and drug-treated cells because any alteration in these parameters would significantly change the measured repair level as represented by the grains per cell value. Fortunately, neither morphine nor cocaine altered thymidine uptake over the range of drug tested in the repair assays and at the concentration of thymidine used in those assays.

Second, phytohemaggluttin-stimulated (PHA) blastogenesis was measured after treatment of the cells with a wide range of morphine concentrations. A significant depression in blastogenesis was found only if the cells were first incubated with the drug for 18 hr. Shorter incubation times were ineffective in impairing blastogenesis, and the presence of the drug in the media throughout the growth phase did not enhance the effectiveness of these shorter incubation times. Thus, the short incubation times (1 hr) which are capable of producing dramatic inhibitions in DNA repair capacity do *not* similarly inhibit DNA synthesis. This suggests that either (1) the opiate block of repair is not linked to the DNA polymerase(s) or deoxynucleoside triphosphates used in DNA synthesis; or (2) the polymerase and/or nucleotides used in the repair process are distinct from (compartmentalized from) those used in blastogenesis. Evidence in the literature is capable of supporting either of these hypotheses.

CAN THE GENETICS OF HUMAN OPIATE ABUSE BE STUDIED IN THE LYMPHOCYTE?

For the above data on the interindividual variability of cellular drug response to be useful in studying the genetics of that response, it must be demonstrated that the interindividual variation is greater than the intraindividual repair variation tested by repeated measurements in a single individual. While this question is still under study, preliminary results have suggested that some individuals show the vigorous, drug-induced enhancement or depression in repair capacity reported here while others show either moderate or no enhancement. This range of responses is well beyond that which we have measured by repeated repair measurements in a small group of subjects. If this trend continues, repair modulation in the human T lymphocyte by drugs of abuse may well prove a useful model in studying the genetics of response to various drugs of abuse. Such studies utilizing results from twin and sibling comparison would be comparatively easy if the model cell is in fact the T lymplocyte as opposed to autopsied CNS tissue. Of course it would be interesting to study the responses of addicted subjects and their near, non-addicted relatives in these assays to see if this response is in any way predictive of addiction.

The DNA repair assays were performed by Curtis Len Chappel and Rodney Mathis and the binding assays by David Ketelsen.

REFERENCES

1. Hiller, JM, Pearson, J, Simon, EJ. Distribution of stereospecific binding of the potent opiate analgesic etorphine in the human brain: Predominance in the limbic system. Res Comm Chem Pathol Pharmacol. 1973; 6:1052-62.

2. Sibinga, NES, Goldstein, A. Opioid peptide and opioid receptors in cells of the immune system. Ann Rev Immunol. 1988; 6:219-249.

3. Madden, JJ, Donahoe, RM. Opiate binding to cells of the immune system. In: Watson, RR, ed. Drugs of abuse and immune function. Boca Raton, CRC Press, 1990 in press.

4. Shavit, Y, Depaulis, A, Martin, FC, Terman, GW, Pechnick, RN, Zane, CJ, Gale, RP, Liebeskind, JC. Involvement of brain opiate receptors in the immune-suppressive effect of morphine. Proc Natl Acad Sci, USA. 1986, 83:7114-17.

5. Wybran, J, Appelboom, T, Famaey, JP, Govaerts, A. Suggestive evidence for receptors for morphine and met-enkephalin on normal human blood T lymphocytes. J Immunol. 1979, 123:1068-72.

6. Mehrishi, JN, Mills, IH. Opiate receptors on lymphocytes and platelets in man. Clin Immunol Immunopathol. 1983, 27:240-6.

7. Madden, JJ, Donahoe, RM, Zwemer-Collins, J, Shafer, D, Falek, A. Binding of naloxone to human T lymphocytes. Biochem Pharmacol. 1987, 36:4103-9.

8. Farrar, WL, Hill, JM, Harel-Bellan, A, Vinocour, M. The immune logical brain. Immunol Rev. 1987, 100:361-78.

9. Mendelsohn, LG, Kerchner, GA, Culwell, M, Ades, EW. Immunoregulation by opioid peptides: absence of classical opioid receptors on human mononuclear cells. J Clin Lab Immunol. 1985, 16:125-30.

10. Carr, DJJ, Bost, KL, Blalock, JE. The production of antibodies which recognize opiate receptors in murine leukocytes. Life Sci. 1988, 42:2615-23.

11. Zozulia, AA, Patsakova, E, Kost, NV. Reaction between endogenous opiates and human peripheral blood lymphocytes. Zhurnal Neuropatologii I Psikhiatrii Imeni SS Korsakova. 1982, 82:60-3.

12. Johnson, HM, Smith, EM, Torres, BA, Blaylock, JE. Regulation of the *in vitro* antibody response by neuroendocrine hormones. Proc Natl Acad Sci, USA. 1982, 79:4171-5.

13. Falek, A, Madden, JJ, Donahoe, RM, Shafer, D. Genetic and immunologic consequences of opiate action on lymphocytes. In: MC Braude & AM Zimmerman, ed. Genetic and perinatal effects of abused substances. New York: Academic Press, 1987:43-68.

14. Shafer, D, Falek, A, Madden, JJ, Tadayon, F, Pline, M, Bokos, PJ, Kuehnle, JC, Mendelson, J. Parallel increases in SCE's at base level and with UV treatment in human opiate users. Mutat Res. 1983, 109:73-82.

15. Madden, JJ, Falek, A, Shafer, D, Glick, JH. Effects of opiates and demographic factors on DNA repair synthesis in human leukocytes. Proc Natl Acad Sci, USA. 1979, 76:5769-73.

16. The recent cold-blooded assassination of Dr. Joseph Wybran as he left his laboratory at Erasmus Hospital in Brussels, Belgium has deprived the field of psychoimmunology of one of its foremost leaders and greatly saddened all of us.

SELECTIVE GUIDE TO CURRENT REFERENCE SOURCES ON TOPICS DISCUSSED IN THIS VOLUME

Behavioral and Biochemical Issues in Substance Abuse

Lynn Kasner Morgan, MLS
James E. Raper, Jr., MSLS

Each issue of *Journal of Addictive Diseases* will feature a section offering suggestions on where to look for further information on topics discussed in the issue. In this volume, our intent is to guide readers to selected sources of current information on behavioral and biochemical issues in substance abuse.

Some published reference sources utilize designated terminology (controlled vocabularies) which must be used to find material on topics of interest. For these a sample of available search terms has been indicated to assist the reader in accessing suitable sources for his/her purposes. Other reference tools use keywords or free-text terms from the title of the document, the abstract and the name of any responsible agency or conference.

Ms. Kasner Morgan is Assistant Professor of Medical Education and Director of the Gustave L. and Janet W. Levy Library of the Mount Sinai Medical Center, Inc. Mr. Raper is Instructor in Medical Education and Technical Services Librarian at Mount Sinai, One Gustave L. Levy Place, New York, NY 10029-6574.

In searching using keywords, be sure to look under all possible synonyms to get at the concept in question.

An asterisk (*) appearing before a published source indicates that all or part of that source is in machine-readable form and can be accessed through an online database search. Database searching is recommended for retrieving sources of information that coordinate multiple variables, concepts or subject areas. Most health sciences libraries offer database services which can include mediated online searching, access to locally mounted datafiles, front-end software packages and CD-ROM technology. Searching can also be done from one's office or home with subscriptions to database services and microcomputers equipped with modems.

Readers are encouraged to consult their librarians for further assistance before undertaking research on a topic.

Suggestions regarding the content and organization of this section are welcome and should be sent to the authors.

1. INDEXING AND ABSTRACTING SOURCES

Place of publication, publisher, start date, frequency of publication, and brief descriptions are noted.

**Biological Abstracts* (1926-) and *Biological Abstracts/RRM* (v.18, 1980-). Philadelphia, BioSciences Information Service, semimonthly. Reports on worldwide research in the life sciences.

See: Concept headings for abstracts, such as behavioral biology, developmental biology-embryology, pharmacology, public health, and toxicology sections.

See: Keyword-in-context subject index.

**Chemical Abstracts*. Columbus, Ohio, American Chemical Society, 1907- , weekly. A key to the world's literature of chemistry and chemical engineering, including journal articles, patents, reviews, technical reports, monographs, conference proceedings, symposia, dissertations, and books.

See: *Index Guide* for cross-referencing and indexing policies.

See: *General Subject Index* terms, such as alcoholic beverages; development, mammalian; drug dependence: drug-drug interactions; drug tolerance: genetics; opiates and opiods; tobacco smoke and smoking.

See: Keyword subject indexes.

**Dissertation Abstracts International. Section B. The Sciences and Engineering*. Ann Arbor, Mich., University Microfilms, v.30, 1969/70- , monthly. Includes author-prepared abstracts of doctoral dissertations from 500 participating institutions throughout North America and the world. A separate section contains European dissertations.

See: Keyword subject index.

**Excerpta Medica*. Amsterdam, The Netherlands, Excerpta Medica Foundation, 1947- , 45 subject sections. A major abstracting service covering more than 4,300 biomedical journals. The abstracts, including English summaries for non-English-language articles, appear in one or more of the published sections, excluding Section 37, *Drug Literature Index*, and Section 38, *Adverse Reactions Titles*, which are indexes only. Each of the sections has a comprehensive subject index. Since 1978 all the *Excerpta Medica* sections have been available for computer searching in the integrated online file, EMBASE.

Particularly relevant to the topics in this issue are Section 8. *Neurology and Neurosurgery*; Section 22, *Human Genetics*; Section 40, *Drug Dependence, Alcohol Abuse and Alcoholism* and the sections that have addiction, alcoholism or drug subdivisions: Section 130, Clinical Pharmacology; Section 30; *Pharmacology*; Section 32, *Psychiatry*; and Section 17, *Public Health, Social Medicine and Epidemiology*.

**Index Medicus* (includes *Bibliography of Medical Reviews*). Bethesda, Md., National Library of Medicine, 1960- , monthly, with annual cumulations. Published as author and subject indexes to more than 3,800 journals in the biomedical sciences. Subject headings are based on the controlled vocabulary or thesaurus, Medical Subject Headings (MeSH). Since 1966 it has been produced from the MEDLARS database, which provides more comprehensive retrieval, including keyword access and English-language abstracts, than its printed counterparts: *Index Medicus*, *International Nursing Index* and *Index to Dental Literature*. As an example of enhanced online retrieval, the check tag "animal" can be coordinated with MeSH to search animal studies.

See: MeSH terms, such as alcohol, ethyl; alcoholism; amphetamines; analgesics: cocaine; diazepam; drug hypersensitivity; drug resistance; genetics; genetics, behavioral; genetics, biochemical; narcotics; nicotine; receptors, endorphin; smoking; substance abuse: substance dependence; substance use disorders.

Index to Scientific Reviews. Philadelphia, Institute for Scientific Information, 1974- , semiannual.

See: Permuterm keyword subject index.

See: Citation index.

**International Pharmaceutical Abstracts*. Washington, D.C., American Society of Hospital Pharmacists, 1964- , semimonthly. A key to the world's literature of pharmacy.

See: IPA subject terms, such as alcoholism, central nervous system drugs, central nervous system stimulants. cocaine, dependence, diazepam, drug abuse, genetics, nicotine, opiates, smoking.

**Psychological Abstracts*. Washington, D.C., American Psychological Association, 1927- , monthly. A compilation of nonevaluative summaries of the world's literature in psychology and related disciplines.

See: Index terms, such as addiction, alcoholism, central nervous system disorders, cocaine, diazepam, drug abuse, drug addiction, drug dependency, drug interactions, drug usage, genetics, nicotine, opiates, tobacco smoking.

**Public Affairs Information Service Bulletin*. New York, Public Affairs Information Service, v.55, 1969- , semimonthly. An index to library material in the field of public affairs and public policy published throughout the world.

See: PAIS subject headings, such as alcoholism, cocaine, drug abuse, drug addicts, drugs, genetic research, narcotics, smoking.

**Science Citation Index*. Philadelphia, Institute for Scientific Information, 1961- , bimonthly.

See: Permuterm keyword subject index.

See: Citation index.

**Social Work Research and Abstracts*. New York, National Association of Social Workers, v.13, 1977- , quarterly.

See: Fields of service sections, such as developmental disabilities/mental retardation, substance use and abuse/alcoholism.

See: Subject index.

**Sociological Abstracts*. San Diego, Calif., Sociological Abstracts, Inc., 1952 - , 5 times per year. A collection of nonevaluative abstracts which reflects the world's serial literature in sociology and related disciplines.

See: *Thesaurus of Sociological Indexing Terms*.

See: Descriptors such as alcohol use, alcoholism, drug abuse, drug addiction, drug use, genetics, opiates, smoking, substance abuse.

2. CURRENT AWARENESS PUBLICATIONS

**Current Contents: Clinical Medicine*. Philadelphia, Institute for Scientific Information, v.15, 1987- , weekly.

See: Keyword index.

**Current Contents: Life Sciences*. Philadelphia, Institute for Scientific Information, v.10, 1967- , weekly.

See: Keyword index.

**Current Contents: Social & Behavioral Sciences*. Philadelphia, Institute for Scientific Information, v.6, 1974- , weekly.

See: Keyword index.

3. BOOKS

Andrews, Theodora. *A Bibliography of Drug Abuse, Including Alcohol and Tobacco*. Littleton, Colo., Libraries Unlimited, 1977- .

Andrews, Theodora. *Guide to the Literature of Pharmacy and the Pharmaceutical Sciences*. Littleton, Colo., Libraries Unlimited, 1986.

**Bibliography on Smoking and Health*. Rockville, Md., Centers for Disease Control, Center for Health Promotion and Education, Office on Smoking and Health, Technical Information Center, 1958/63- , annual.

Cocaine: An Annotated Bibliography. Jackson, Research Institute of Pharmaceutical Sciences, University of Mississippi and University Press of Mississippi, c1988.

**Medical and Health Care Books and Serials in Print: An Index to Literature in the Health Sciences*. New York, R. R. Bowker Co., annual.

See: Library of Congress subject headings, such as alcohol, amphetamines, behavior genetics, cocaine, drug abuse, drugs, genetics, laboratory animals, narcotic habit, smoking.

**National Library of Medicine Current Catalog*. Bethesda, Md., National Library of Medicine, 1966- , quarterly, with annual cumulations.

See: MeSH terms as noted in Section 1 under *Index Medicus*.

Page, Penny B. *Alcohol Use and Alcoholism: A Guide to the Literature*. New York, Garland Publishing, 1986.

World Health Organization Catalogue: New Books. Geneva, World Health Organization, semiannual (supplements *World Health Organization Publications* and includes periodicals).

4. U.S. GOVERNMENT PUBLICATIONS

**Monthly Catalog of United States Government Publications*. Washington, D.C., U.S. Government Printing Office, 1895- , monthly.

See: Following agencies: Alcohol, Drug Abuse and Mental Health Administration: Food and Drug Administration: National Institute of Mental Health: National Institute on Drug Abuse; National Institutes of Health; U.S. Dept. of Agriculture.

See: Subject headings, derived chiefly from the Library of Congress, such as alcohol; amphetamines; alcoholism; behavior genetics; cocaine; drug abuse; drug utilization; drug dependence; drugs: genetics: genetics, biochemical: laboratory animals; narcotics: opiods; psychopharmacology.

See: Title index.

5. ONLINE BIBLIOGRAPHIC DATABASES

Only those databases which have no print equivalents are included in this section. Print sources which have online database equivalents are noted throughout this guide by the asterisk (*) which appears before the title. If you do not have direct access to these databases, consult your librarian for assistance.

ALCOHOL AND ALCOHOL PROBLEMS SCIENCE DATABASE (National Institute on Alcohol Abuse and Alcoholism, Rockville, Md.).

Use: Keywords.

ALCOHOL INFORMATION FOR CLINICIANS AND EDUCATORS (Project Cork Institute, Dartmouth Medical School, Hanover, N.H.)

Use: Keywords.

ASI: AMERICAN STATISTICS INDEX (Congressional Information Services, Inc., Washington, D.C.).

Use: Keywords.

DRUG INFORMATION FULLTEXT (American Society of Hospital Pharmacists, Bethesda, Md.)

Use: Keywords

DRUGINFO AND ALCOHOL USE AND ABUSE (Hazelden Foundation, Center City, Minn. and Drug Information Service Center, College of Pharmacy, University of Minnesota, Minneapolis, Minn.).

Use: Keywords.

FAMILY RESOURCES DATABASE (National Council on Family Relations and Inventory of Marriage and Family Literature Project, Minneapolis, Minn.).

Use: Keywords.

LEXIS (Mead Data Central, Inc., Dayton, OH).

Use: Keywords.

MAGAZINE INDEX (Information Access Co., Belmont, Calif.).

Use: Keywords.

MEDICAL AND PSYCHOLOGICAL PREVIEWS: MPPS (BRS Bibliographic Retrieval Services, Inc., McLean, Va.).

Use: Keywords.

MENTAL HEALTH ABSTRACTS (IFI/Plenum Data Co., Alexandria, Va.).

Use: Keywords.

NATIONAL NEWSPAPER INDEX (Information Access Co., Belmont, Calif.).

Use: Keywords.

NTIS (National Technical Information Service, U.S. Dept. of Commerce, Springfield, Va.).

Use: Keywords.

PSYCALERT (American Psychological Association, Washington, D.C.).

Use: Keywords.

WESTLAW (West Publishing Co., St. Paul, Minn.)

Use: Keywords.

6. HANDBOOKS, DIRECTORIES, GRANT SOURCES, ETC.

Annual Register of Grant Support. Wilmette, Ill., National Register Pub. Co., annual.

See: Biology; medicine; neurology; pharmacology; psychiatry, psychology, mental health sections.

See: Subject index.

Biomedical Index to PHA-Supported Research. Bethesda, Md., National Institutes of Health, Division of Research Grants, annual.

See: Subject index.

**Database Directory*. White Plains, N.Y., Knowledge Industry Publications in cooperation with the American Society for Information Science, annual.

See: Subject Index.

**Directory of Online Databases* (includes *Online Databases in the Medical and Life Sciences*). New York, Cuadra/Elsevier, quarterly.

See: Subject Index

Directory of Research Grants. Phoenix, Az., Oryx Press, annual.

See: Subject index terms, such as alcoholism, drug abuse.

**Encyclopedia of Associations*. Detroit, Gale Research Co., annual (occasional supplements between editions).

See: Subject index.

Encyclopedia of Information Systems and Services. Detroit, Gale Research Co., annual.

**Foundation Directory*. New York, The Foundation Center, biennial (updated between editions by *Foundation Directory Supplement*).

See: Index of foundations.

See: Index of foundations by state and city.

See: Index of donors, trustees and administrators.

See: Index of fields of interest.

O'Brien, Robert and Sidney Cohen. *The Encyclopedia of Drug Abuse*. New York, Facts on File Pub., 1984.

Roper, Fred W. and Jo Anne Boorkman. *Introduction to Reference Sources in the Health Sciences*. 2nd ed. Chicago, Medical Library Association, © 1984.

The SALIS Directory: Substance Abuse Librarians and Information Specialists. Berkeley, Calif., Alcohol Research Group, Medical Research Institute of San Francisco and University of California, Berkeley, 1987-88, © 1987.

Statistics Sources. Detroit, Gale Research Co., annual.

7. JOURNAL LISTINGS

**Ulrich's International Periodicals Directory, Now Including Irregular Serials & Annuals*. New York, R. R. Bowker Co., annual (updated between editions by *Ulrich's Quarterly*).

See: Subject categories, such as biology, drug abuse and alcoholism, medical sciences, pharmacy and pharmacology, tobacco.

8. AUDIOVISUAL PROGRAMS

**National Library of Medicine Audiovisuals Catalog*. Bethesda. Md., National Library of Medicine, 1977- , quarterly, with annual cumulations.

See: *MeSH* terms as noted in Section 1 under *Index Medicus*.

Patient Education Sourcebook. [Saint Louis, Mo.]. Health Sciences Communications Association, © 1985.

See: *MeSH* terms as noted in Section 1 under *Index Medicus*.

9. GUIDES TO UPCOMING MEETINGS

Scientific Meetings. San Diego, Calif., Scientific Meetings Publications, quarterly.

See: Subject indexes.

See: Association listing.

World Meetings: Medicine. New York, Macmillan Pub. Co., quarterly.

See: Keyword index.

See: Sponsor directory and index.

World Meetings: Outside United States and Canada. New York, Macmillan Pub. Co., quarterly.

See: Keyword index.

See: Sponsor directory and index.

World Meetings: United States and Canada. New York, Macmillan Pub. Co., quarterly.

See: Keyword index.

See: Sponsor directory and index.

10. PROCEEDINGS OF MEETINGS

**Conference Papers Index*. Louisville, Ky., Data Courier, v.6, 1978- , monthly.

Directory of Published Proceedings. Series SEMT. Science/Engineering/Medicine/Technology. White Plains, N.Y., InterDok Corp., v.3, 1967- , monthly, except July-August, with annual cumulations.

**Index to Scientific and Technical Proceedings*. Philadelphia, Institute for Scientific Information, 1978- , monthly with semiannual cumulations.

11. SPECIALIZED RESEARCH CENTERS

Medical Research Centres. 8th ed. Harlow, Essex, Longman, 1988.

International Research Centers Directory. 5th ed. Detroit, Gale Research Co., 1990-91, © 1990.

Research Centers Directory. Detroit, Gale Research Co., annual (updated by *New Research Centers*).

12. SPECIAL LIBRARY COLLECTIONS

Ash, L., comp. *Subject Collections*. 6th ed. New York, R. R. Bowker Co., 1985.

Directory of Special Libraries and Information Centers. 13th ed. Detroit, Gale Research Co., 1990 (updated by *New Special Libraries*).

For Product Safety Concerns and Information please contact our EU representative GPSR@taylorandfrancis.com Taylor & Francis Verlag GmbH, Kaufingerstraße 24, 80331 München, Germany